Radiology
FOR THE MRCP

Commissioning Editor: Laurence Hunter
Project Development Manager: Jim Killgore
Project Manager: Fiona Young
Designer: Erik Bigland

Radiology
FOR THE MRCP

Jeremy Hughes MA MRCP PhD
Wellcome Trust Advanced Fellow and Visiting Scholar,
University of Washington, Seattle, USA

Michael Hughes FRCSEd FRCR
Consultant Radiologist, Postgraduate Clinical Tutor,
Warwick Hospital, Warwick, UK

Iain D Lyburn MRCP(UK) FRCR
Fellow in Abdominal Imaging, Vancouver General Hospital,
Vancouver, Canada

Foreword by
Professor John Savill BA MB ChB FRCP FmedSci
Professor of Medicine, University of Edinburgh
Edinburgh, UK

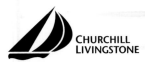
CHURCHILL
LIVINGSTONE

EDINBURGH LONDON NEW YORK PHILADELPHIA ST LOUIS SYDNEY TORONTO 2000

CHURCHILL LIVINGSTONE
An imprint of Harcourt Publishers Limited

First published 2000

ISBN 0443 06041 X

**British Library Cataloguing in Publication
Data**
A catalogue record for this book is available
from the British Library

**Library of Congress Cataloging in
Publication Data**
A catalog record for this book is available from
the Library of Congress

Note
Medical knowledge is constantly changing. As
new information becomes available, changes
in treatment, procedures, equipment and the
use of drugs become necessary. The authors
and the publishers have, as far as it is possible,
taken care to ensure that the information given
in this text is accurate and up to date.
However, readers are strongly advised to
confirm that the information, especially with
regard to drug usage, complies with the latest
legislation and standards of practice.

Printed in China

FOREWORD

When interpreting investigations in the context of the clinical problem posed by a patient, the best physicians always examine the primary data. In particular, the physician should be able to make a preliminary assessment of relevant radiological investigations, whilst remembering that the full yield of information will only emerge when the expert opinion of the radiologist is available and is discussed. For these reasons radiology features, very properly, in the MRCP(UK) examination. However, few post-MRCP physicians will forget the anxiety provoked during this ordeal by the unheralded appearance of an apparently normal chest X-ray. This excellent book will go a long way towards banishing such anxiety, and will give any physician increased confidence in interpreting a wide range of radiological investigations, including CT, MRI, contrast studies and isotope scans. Indeed, the work also serves as an excellent revision text for much of medicine. However, I do have one recommendation – if you lend this book to a colleague, make sure you get it back!

Professor John Savill
2000

This book is primarily intended for medical postgraduates preparing for the MRCP examination but enthusiastic medical students may also find it useful and informative. Our aim is to test the reader's powers of observation, deduction and interpretation, as well as basic medical knowledge of the various specialties, which is a necessary prerequisite to passing the rigorous MRCP examination. We also hope that after successfully passing the MRCP examination the reader will continue to enjoy studying the images derived from radiological investigations undergone by their patients, for the old adage of 'a picture can tell a thousand words' applies equally in radiology as in clinical medicine.

J.H.   2000
M. H.
I.D.L.

ACKNOWLEDGEMENTS

This book is dedicated to our parents, wives (Brenda [JH], Caroline [MH] and Sonia [IL]) and children (Lloyd, Owen and Rhian [JH]; Charlotte, Rebecca and Edward [MH] and Eleanor [IL]) for their patience and encouragement during the preparation of this book.

We are grateful to Dr M. P. Callaway, Dr V. N. Cassar-Pullicino, Ms L. Cheney, Dr M. Darby, Dr M. Griffiths, Professor J. R. Hampton, Dr T. S. I. Lyburn, Professor I. W. McCall, Dr M. Roberts, Professor P. C. Ruben, Dr S. D. Ryder and Dr J. Virjee for permission to use their radiographs. MH would also like to thank his clinical and departmental colleagues at Warwick Hospital. Further help from Alliance Medical Ltd, for assistance with some of the MRI scan cases, and from staff at Leamington Camera Exchange, for regular expert photographic advice, is also much appreciated.

CONTENTS

ABDOMEN AND PELVIS

Introduction: abdomen and pelvis

The abdomen and pelvis can be assessed utilising all the modalities in imaging: plain radiographs, contrast studies (see Section 3), ultrasound, computed tomography (CT) magnetic resonance imaging (MRI) and nuclear medicine.

A plain radiograph is a two-dimensional representation of a three-dimensional object — further assessment of complex structures can be made by CT and MRI (cross sectional imaging) as the problem of overlapping structures is effectively eliminated. Ultrasound is relatively inexpensive, does not expose the patient to ionising radiation and may be performed portably, i.e. at the patient's bedside; disadvantages include its inability to penetrate gas-containing structures (e.g. bowel) and bone, in addition to decreased resolution with depth, making the investigation of obese patients difficult.

Non-radiologists are required to be able to interpret plain radiographs, as often further management decisions will be based upon these interpretations prior to formal reporting of the film by a radiologist. In the usual clinical setting more complex examinations are reported by radiologists; for diploma examination purposes candidates should be familiar with the appearance of certain conditions.

When looking at a plain abdominal radiograph observe:

- The way the film was taken (erect, supine or decubitus; inspiration or expiration). Free gas and fluid levels are apparent on erect films.

- Region covered. This should include the diaphragm above and femoral canals below.

- Luminal gas pattern and distribution. The small bowel valvulae conniventes traverse the bowel lumen and small bowel loops tend to lie in the centre of the abdomen. Haustral folds of the large bowel traverse about one third of the lumen diameter and the loops tend to be peripheral.

- Extraluminal gas. The presence of a gas shadow which does not conform to a bowel loop should raise the suspicion that gas lies in the intraperitoneal space, suggestive of a perforation, be it in a retroperitoneal location or in a viscus that does not usually contain gas, such as the biliary tree.

- Thickness of the bowel mucosa, valvulae conniventes and haustra.

- Areas of calcification. These include vascular (parallel lines, curvilinear if related to an aneurysm), phleboliths (circular with lucent centre), lymph nodes (irregular granular opacities), gallstones (concentric faceted rings), renal calculi (constantly related to renal outline as shown on inspiration compared with expiration film; if in ureter shown on intravenous urogram), bladder (calculi or related to wall), fibroids (nodular conglomerations), suprarenal (triangular related to upper kidney), pancreatic (line of pancreas from right of L1/L2 upwards and left to hilum of spleen), hepatic and splenic.

- Organ outlines and displacement. Look for enlargement of liver, spleen and kidneys, or displaced loops of bowel.

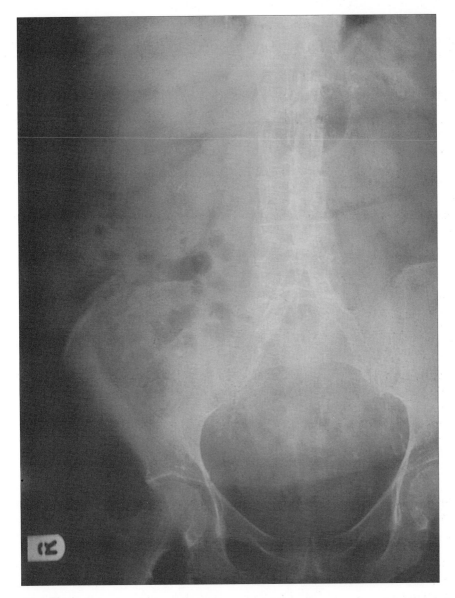

This abdominal X-ray is of a 76-year-old woman who developed renal failure after beginning treatment for congestive cardiac failure.

A Describe the abnormality.
B Suggest what treatment she was given and why she developed renal failure.
C What treatment is required?

[A] There is marked calcification of the aorta and main vessels.

[B] The patient had begun taking an angiotensin-converting enzyme (ACE) inhibitor. She developed renal failure as she had atheromatous bilateral renal artery stenosis.

[C] Treatment consists of immediate cessation of the ACE inhibitor together with supportive treatment for the renal failure; this may include acute dialysis, although renal function may well not recover in this context.

Elderly patients who are about to start taking ACE inhibitors for hypertension or congestive cardiac failure should be examined for clinical evidence of significant vascular disease as, if this is present, they may well have underlying renal artery atheromatous disease. It is therefore important to look for vascular calcification on the patients' X-rays. This patient has marked atheromatous vascular disease and such patients should be assumed to have atheromatous renovascular disease, possibly bilateral, until proved otherwise, particularly if they have renal impairment. These patients may require further imaging with MRI, spiral CT scanning or intra-arterial renal angiography (Fig. 1.1.1), although the latter investigation may be complicated by contrast nephropathy, cholesterol emboli or dissection of the arterial wall. Plain X-rays may also reveal other important pathology such as aneurysmal dilatation of large vessels (Fig. 1.1.2, arrow).

Arterial calcification

- Diabetes (esp. digital vessels)
- Atheromatous disease
- Chronic renal failure (esp. elevated Ca/PO_4 product)
- Hyperlipidaemia
- Hyperparathyroidism

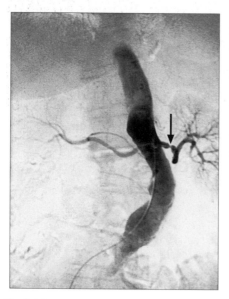

Fig. 1.1.1

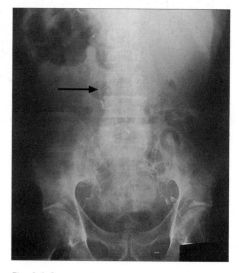

Fig. 1.1.2

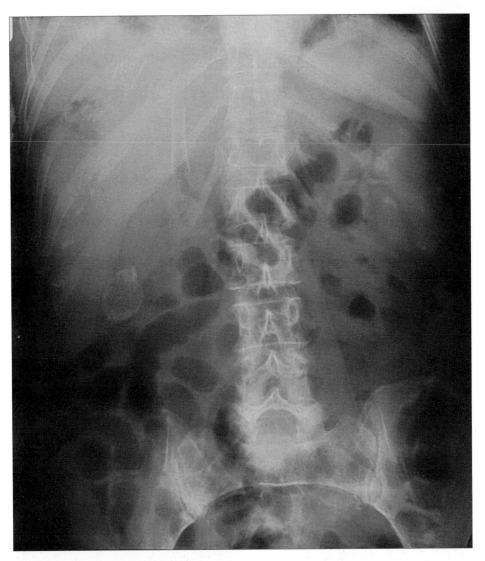

This abdominal X-ray is of a 64-year-old woman who has become unwell after treatment for jaundice.

A What treatment has been performed?
B What complication has occurred?
C What treatment is required?

A A metallic wall stent has been inserted into the biliary tree and can be seen just to the right of the lower thoracic vertebrae. In addition there is a porcelain gall bladder, aerobilia and a collection of gas overlying the right lobe of the liver.

B This patient has developed a suppurative ascending cholangitis complicated by the development of a hepatic abscess.

C Treatment consists of general supportive measures, percutaneous drainage of the abscess under ultrasound or CT guidance and broad spectrum intravenous antibiotics.

The presence of gas in the soft tissues is an extremely important radiological sign. The gas in this case overlies the liver, is obviously separate from the gas within the bowel and is strongly suggestive of a hepatic abscess. An abscess may be confirmed by ultra-sound (Fig. 1.2.1) or CT scanning (Fig. 1.2.2). Indeed this patient had multiple abscesses requiring imaging-guided drainage (Fig. 1.2.3; note contrast outlining abscess cavity).

Aerobilia is not an uncommon radiological finding and is usually secondary to instrumentation of the biliary system but may also be the consequence of a fistula between the gall bladder or bile duct and the stomach or duodenum resulting from gallstones, tumours or penetrating peptic ulcer disease.

Causes of a focal low attenuation lesion(s) in the liver on unenhanced CT include pyogenic abscess, amoebic abscess (*Entamoeba histolytica*), hydatid disease (*Echinococcus granulosus* or *multilocularis*), fungal abscess (usually small and multiple), simple cyst, polycystic liver disease, cavernous haemangioma as well as primary hepatocellular carcinoma or metastatic carcinoma.

Causes of gas in biliary system (i.e. aerobilia)
• Instrumentation (e.g. ERCP)
• Related to surgery (e.g. choledochoduodenostomy)
• Biliary fistulae
• Patulous sphincter of Oddi (elderly)

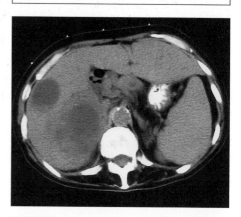

Fig. 1.2.2

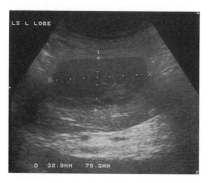

Fig. 1.2.1

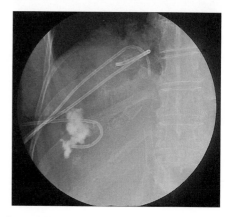

Fig. 1.2.3

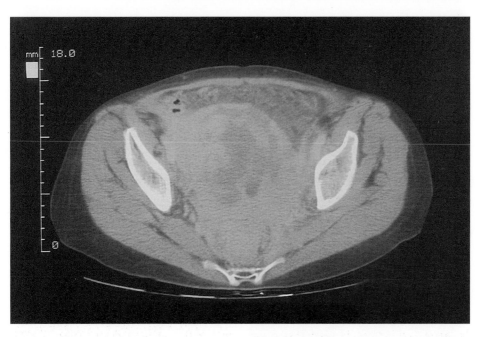

This image from a non-contrast abdominal/pelvic CT scan is of a 52-year-old woman who was admitted with advanced renal impairment. She had received chemotherapy for acute myeloid leukaemia 12 months earlier, which resulted in a clinical remission.

A Describe the abnormality.
B Suggest an underlying diagnosis and a cause for her renal failure.
C What treatment is required?

A A very large mixed attenuation pelvic mass is evident.

B In view of the history of recent acute myeloid leukaemia (AML) this mass may well be a chloroma. A peculiar feature of AML is that leukaemic blast cells may accumulate to form a rapidly growing mass and this can occur in any tissue. Renal failure in the context of a large pelvic tumour is most likely to be secondary to bilateral ureteric obstruction.

C Treatment consists of the insertion of bilateral nephrostomies (with platelet cover if necessary) and careful fluid and electrolyte balance. Further chemotherapy should be considered as chloromas may well be chemotherapy sensitive.

There are numerous causes of pelvic tumours, including benign and malignant ovarian tumours (Fig. 1.3.1, note large rounded pelvic opacity), uterine fibroids and carcinoma of the bladder, prostate, cervix and colon.

Obstructive renal failure

● Tumours of urinary tract (bladder and prostate)

● Extrinsic malignant obstruction (cervix and colon)

● Stone-related disease (esp. with solitary or single functioning kidney)

● Retroperitoneal fibrosis (Fig. 1.3.2)

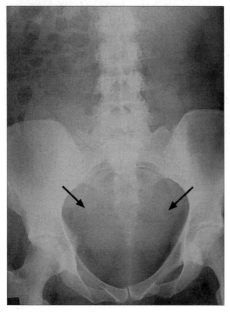

Fig. 1.3.1

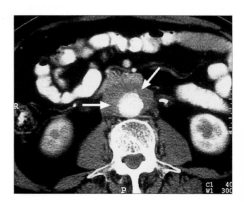

Fig. 1.3.2

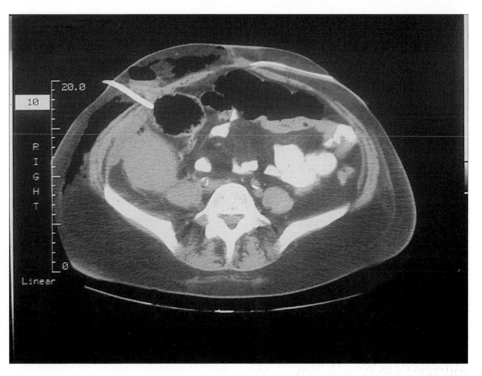

This abdominal CT scan is of a 46-year-old woman who developed an intra-abdominal urinoma (collection of urine) after a cadaveric renal transplant that required percutaneous drainage.

A Describe the abnormality and suggest two predisposing factors.
B What clinical signs may be present?
C What treatment is required?

A The renal transplant is evident in the right iliac fossa with the drain lying anteriorly. There is a large collection of gas and some fluid in the right anterior abdominal wall indicative of sepsis with gas-forming bacteria. Predisposing factors include the post-transplant immuno-suppressive drug regimen, pre-existing (or steroid-induced) diabetes mellitus and a potential track of infection along the drainage tube.

B The patient may be systemically un-well, although a fever may be absent or mild (secondary to immunosuppression). Abdominal signs may include localized tenderness, erythema and surgical crepitus.

C Treatment consists of high-dose intra-venous antibiotics after multiple cultures of blood and urine (MSU/CSU and urine draining from the urinoma). If the patient does not improve clinically then surgical intervention will be required.

The presence of gas within the abdomen but outside the bowel lumen is an important radiological sign. It may represent perforation of an abdominal viscus or infection with a gas-forming organism, either of which requires prompt recognition and institution of treatment. Gas may be within an organ such as in a liver, pancreatic or renal abscess (Fig. 1.4.1) or outside as in a subphrenic abscess. Some conditions such as emphysematous chole-cystitis (Fig. 1.4.2, gas in gall bladder wall) occur more commonly in patients with poorly controlled diabetes mellitus. Extra-luminal gas may also be evident on plain X-rays in pneumatosis intestinalis (Fig. 1.4.3, gas in bowel wall), which may be secondary to chronic obstructive pulmonary disease, necrotizing enterocolitis or mesenteric vascular disease.

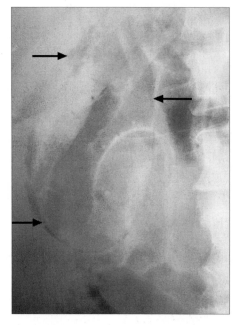

Fig. 1.4.2

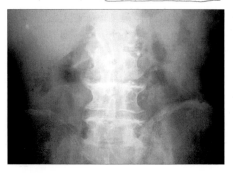

Fig. 1.4.1

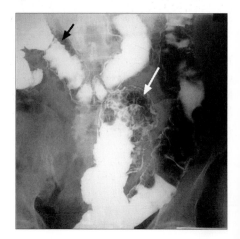

Fig. 1.4.3

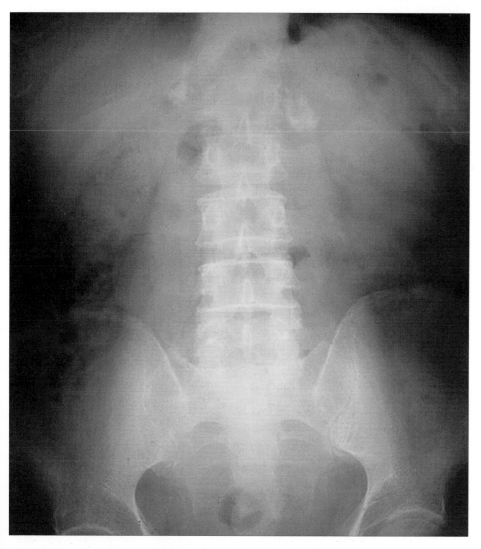

This plain abdominal X-ray is from a 22-year-old man who was admitted to hospital feeling generally unwell with weakness and lethargy. Investigations revealed the following levels: sodium 120 mmol/L, potassium 7.2 mmol/L, urea 9.6 mmol/L and creatinine 100 µmol/L.

A Describe the abnormality and suggest a diagnosis and underlying cause.
B What is the cause of the biochemical disturbance?
C What treatment is required?

A There is bilateral adrenal calcification. The history, X-ray appearance and biochemistry indicates adrenocortical insufficiency (Addison's disease). This case was secondary to tuberculosis.

B Aldosterone stimulates the retention of sodium in exchange for potassium in the distal tubules and therefore potassium is retained in hypoaldosteronaemic states. The loss of sodium and accompanying water leads to hypovolaemia, hypotension and hyponatraemia.

C This patient requires urgent correction of the hyperkalaemia (cardioprotective i.v. calcium and i.v. dextrose and insulin) together with intravenous fluids. A synacthen test will confirm the diagnosis and the patient will require lifelong replacement therapy with hydrocortisone and fludrocortisone.

Adrenocortical failure can be caused by a wide range of pathologies, only some of which result in adrenal calcification. In 60% of patients, the adrenocortical failure is idiopathic (probably autoimmune re-lated). Additional causes include granulomatous disease (TB as in this patient) or sarcoidosis. Infective causes include fungi (e.g. histoplasmosis or coccidioidomycosis).

Intra-adrenal haemorrhage (neonates, coagulopathies or sepsis), if it involves more than 90% of the adrenal cortex, will usually result in permanent adrenal insuffiency.

Bilateral adrenal metastatic disease should be actively excluded in patients with a known history of malignant disease (esp. bronchial primary tumours) (Fig. 1.5.1).

Differentiate from other more common causes of upper abdominal calcification evident on plain abdominal X-rays (e.g. chronic pancreatitis, gallstones and renal calculi).

Causes of adrenal calcification
● Tuberculosis
● Neonatal adrenal haemorrhage
● Cystic adrenal disease (15% are bilateral)
● Tumours (neuroblastomas and phaeochromocytomas)

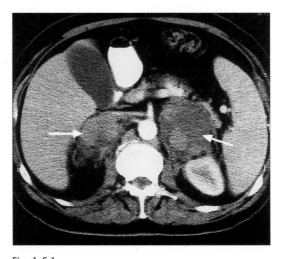

Fig. 1.5.1

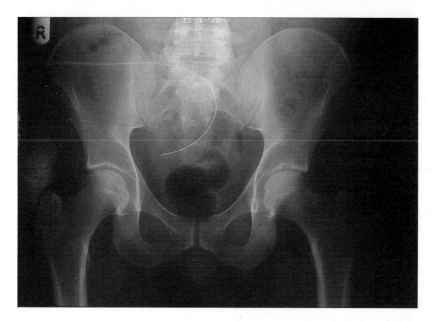

This X-ray is of a 48-year-old man.

A Describe two abnormalities that are visible.
B Suggest two different possible diagnoses.

ANSWER 1.6

A There is an indwelling abdominal Tenchkoff catheter for chronic ambulatory peritoneal dialysis (CAPD) together with a calcified mass in the soft tissues lateral to the right greater trochanter.

B This patient has end-stage renal failure, which may be secondary to a myriad of causes, and has developed ectopic calcification either as a result of deranged calcium and phosphate balance or in response to the development of tertiary hyperparathyroidism.

Alternatively, the patient may have had primary hyperparathyroidism, which subsequently resulted in renal failure secondary to renal calculi (kidneys not visible on this X-ray) and may also cause ectopic calcification.

Ectopic metastatic calcification of the periarticular and soft tissues may occur in other disorders of calcium and phosphate metabolism, including idiopathic hypercalcaemia, hyperparathyroidism, hypervitaminosis D and the milk alkali syndrome. In hyperparathyroidism the calcific deposits may be dense and massive producing so-called 'tumoral calcinosis' as in Figure 1.6.1 where the axilla is involved. Such cases may require surgery. A similar appearance may occasionally occur in a calcified tophus.

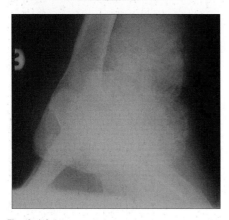

Fig. 1.6.1

Soft-tissue calcification

It is useful to distinguish between the two main groups:

● metastatic (deposition of calcium salts in previously normal tissues – abnormal calcium homeostasis)

● dystrophic (normal systemic calcium metabolism and abnormal local electrolyte/enzyme disturbance e.g. post-traumatic)

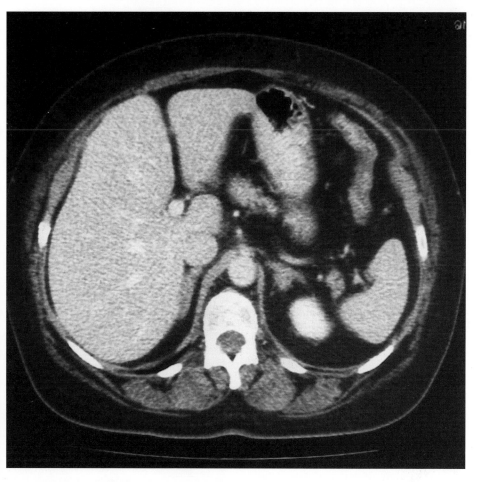

This CT scan (level of section is just above the kidneys) is of a 74-year-old woman who is undergoing investigation for recent onset hypertension and weight gain.

A Describe the abnormality and suggest a diagnosis.
B What clinical and biochemical signs may be present?
C What diagnostic tests are available?

A There is a large enhancing left-sided lesion in the position of the adrenal gland compatible with a left adrenal adenoma (Fig. 1.7.1), although an adrenal carcinoma cannot be excluded. This patient has Cushing's syndrome.

B Clinical signs include central obesity, a buffalo hump, proximal muscle weakness, acne and striae. Biochemical changes include glucose intolerance or frank diabetes mellitus and hypokalaemia.

C A simple screening test is the overnight dexamethasone suppression test. The patient takes 1 mg dexamethasone at 11 pm and at 8 am the following day the serum cortisol is measured. A cortisol level below 5 µg/dL or 138 nmoles/L almost certainly excludes the condition. If abnormal then a 24-hour urine collection should be performed to demonstrate hypercortisolism. An elevated plasma ACTH indicates a pituitary tumour or ectopic secretion, whereas a subnormal ACTH level suggests an adrenal tumour.

The majority of patients (70%) with hypercortisolism have Cushing's disease (ACTH-secreting pituitary adenoma) whereas an adrenal tumour or bilateral hyperplasia is found in about 15%. The remaining patients have a paraneoplastic Cushing's syndrome with ectopic ACTH production, e.g. patients with carcinoma of the bronchus or, less commonly, pancreas, kidney or prostate. Patients with a paraneoplastic Cushing's syndrome often have a severe biochemical disturbance but not the characteristic clinical features (buffalo hump etc.), which take some time to develop although hyperpigmentation is common. An adrenal adenoma may be difficult to distinguish from an adrenal carcinoma on CT scan. Clinical evidence of virilization would suggest a carcinoma. In bilateral hyperplasia the glands, though enlarged, retain their characteristic triangular shape. In Cushing's disease, about 50% of patients have a detectable pituitary adenoma on MRI scan. Patients with Cushing's syndrome may develop osteoporosis.

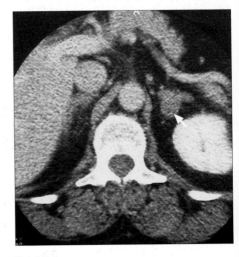

Fig. 1.7.1

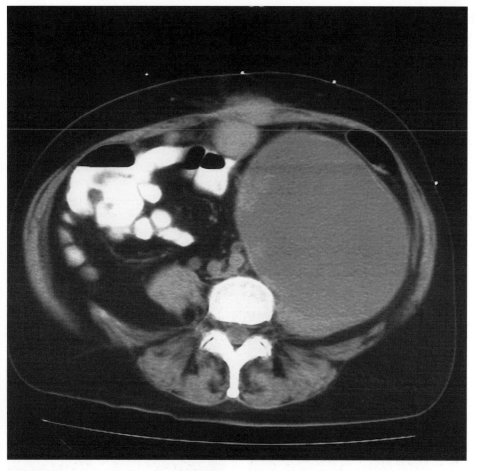

This CT scan is of a 55-year-old woman who was referred to hospital with an 'umbilical hernia'. On examination she was found to have a large abdominal mass.

A Describe the abnormalities and suggest a unifying diagnosis.
B What was the umbilical hernia?
C What treatment is available?

A There is a very large left-sided cystic mass. In addition, there are abnormal rounded soft-tissue masses within and just below the central abdominal wall.

B The 'umbilical hernia' is actually a metastatic deposit that is often given the name of Sister Josephine's nodule. It is a reflection of advanced intra-abdominal malignancy (in this case a left ovarian primary lesion).

C Treatment for ovarian cancer consists of surgical removal (e.g. bilateral salpingo-oophorectomy with abdominal hysterectomy, omentectomy and selective lymphadenectomy) followed by postoperative chemotherapy. Cyst decompression (Fig. 1.8.1, same patient following guided pig-tail catheter placement) and abdominocentesis can provide symptom relief.

The presence of a positive family history (first-degree relatives) for ovarian cancer increases the risk of developing an ovarian neoplasm. As early ovarian malignancy is asymptomatic, such high-risk women may be screened with annual transvaginal ultrasound and measurement of the levels of the tumour marker CA 125 (elevated in 50% of patients with early disease). Unfortunately many patients still present with advanced disease with an abdominal mass or malignant ascites (Fig. 1.8.2). Differentiating benign from malignant ovarian masses using ultrasound is at present still controversial.

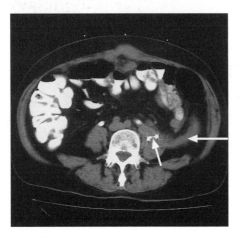

Fig. 1.8.1

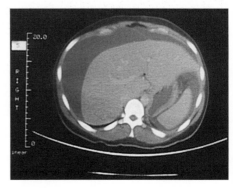

Fig. 1.8.2

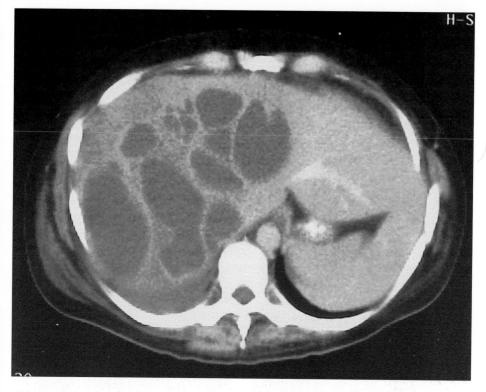

This CT scan is of a 65-year-old man who presented with a pyrexia of unknown origin. He had a long history of mild diverticular disease.

A Describe the abnormality.
B Suggest a diagnosis and treatment.

A There are multiple low attenuation lesions throughout the right lobe of the liver, which are characteristic of abscesses.

B The most likely diagnosis is multiple hepatic abscesses arising as a complication of subclinical diverticulitis. Treatment involves percutaneous drainage under ultrasound or CT guidance (Fig. 1.9.1) with culture of aspirated pus combined with broad spectrum antibiotics (third-generation cephalosporin and metronidazole). Small abscesses may not require drainage if a rapid clinical response follows antibiotic treatment.

The patient's diverticular disease must be assessed when he is clinically fit.

Bacteria may spread to the liver via the portal vein (pyelophlebitis), hepatic artery (bacteraemia), common bile duct (ascending cholangitis) or directly from an adjacent infective focus. The commonest cause in tropical and subtropical regions is an amoebic abscess. In the UK the commonest cause is biliary disease (obstruction secondary to gallstones, stricture or tumours) followed by diverticulitis and appendicitis. Many abscesses are cryptogenic and have no identifiable cause.

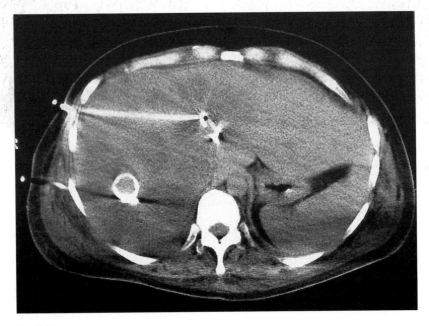

Fig. 1.9.1

QUESTION 1.10

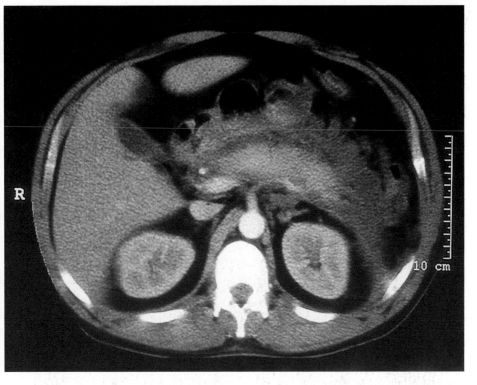

This CT scan is of a 40-year-old man who was admitted to hospital with acute abdominal pain.

A Describe the abnormality and suggest a diagnosis.
B Give two predisposing causes.
C Outline potential complications and treatment.

ANSWER 1.10

A The pancreas is grossly abnormal with marked swelling and retroperitoneal oedema. This patient has severe acute pancreatitis.

B The commonest predisposing causes are alcohol and biliary calculus disease. Other causes include hyperlipidaemia, viral infections (e.g. mumps), drugs and abdominal trauma or instrumentation (ERCP).

C Local complications include the development of a pseudocyst or an abscess. Patients typically develop a paralytic ileus, and intravascular volume depletion may result in severe hypotension or even acute tubular necrosis.

Further complications include the adult respiratory distress syndrome, particularly if patients have required large volumes of intravenous fluid and colloid. In the long term up to 10% of cases are complicated by chronic pancreatitis with the development of pancreatic exocrine insufficiency and diabetes mellitus.

Treatment primarily consists of nil by mouth, nasogastric suction, analgesia and intravenous fluids. Antibiotics are indicated when infection is documented or highly suspected. Total parenteral nutrition may be necessary if the ileus is prolonged.

Surgery is indicated in patients with marked necrosis or infection. Abscesses and pseudocysts may require imaging-guided drainage.

Imaging can be informative in patients with acute abdominal pain although the presence of gallstones on a plain abdominal film does not indicate that they are the cause of the symptoms! A pneumoperitoneum with gas under the diaphragm indicates perforation of an intra-abdominal viscus (Fig. 1.10.1). This may be clinically silent in the elderly when patients present with non-specific symptoms. The loss of hepatic dullness can be a useful clinical sign in this context. In pancreatitis the abdominal X-ray may demonstrate a sentinel loop whereas the chest X-ray may exhibit basal atelectasis or a pleural effusion, which is most commonly left sided. Ultrasound and CT are useful for monitoring patients and the early detection of local complications.

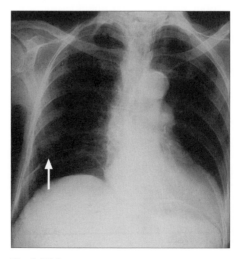

Fig. 1.10.1

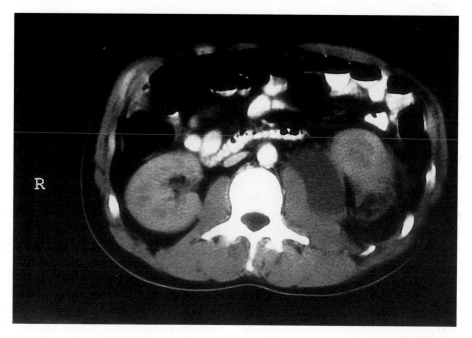

This CT scan is of a 45-year-old man who is on warfarin treatment after a prosthetic heart valve procedure. He was admitted to hospital with severe flank pain.

A. Describe the abnormality and suggest a diagnosis.

B. Suggest a potential cause and outline treatment.

A The left retroperitoneum is abnormal, with a large homogenous mass that is displacing the left kidney. In view of the history of anticoagulation the most likely diagnosis is retroperitoneal bleeding with formation of a haematoma.

B Predisposing causes include incorrect dosing with warfarin or ingestion of drugs that potentiate the anticoagulant action of warfarin.

Retroperitoneal haemorrhage is sometimes seen in patients who are overtreated with warfarin. Another group of patients who are at risk of this complication are those treated with systemic thrombolytic agents (most commonly acute myocardial infarction patients).

CT scanning is very useful for scrutinizing the retroperitoneum (which can be difficult to visualize by ultrasound because of the presence of gas-filled bowel loops) in conditions such as iliopsoas haemorrhage (Fig. 1.11.1).

MRI scanning is also utilized extensively; e.g. Figure 1.11.2 demonstrates an early left psoas abscess as an extension of an infective discitis.

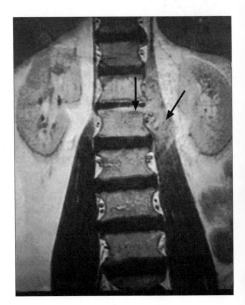

Fig. 1.11.2

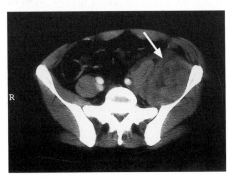

Fig. 1.11.1

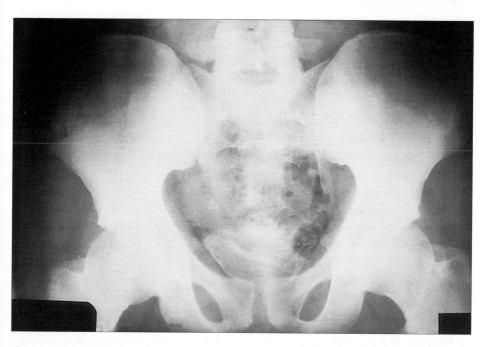

This plain pelvic X-ray is of a 29-year-old man with recurrent haematuria.

A   Describe the abnormality and suggest a cause.
B   What further investigation is required?
C   Outline treatment.

[A] There is spectacular calcification of the bladder with a dilated calcified left distal ureter. The underlying diagnosis is chronic infection with schistosomiasis (*schistosoma haematobium*).

[B] A cystoscopy should be performed to exclude a complicating bladder carcinoma.

[C] Antihelminthic treatment with praziquantel results in an almost 90% cure rate although reinfection may occur.

Schistosomiasis is the commonest cause of bladder calcification worldwide. The infestation results in a granulomatous inflammatory reaction. There is an increased incidence of squamous cell carcinoma in these patients. Genitourinary tuberculosis may cause calcification of the distal ureter but, in contrast to renal tuberculosis, calcification of the bladder is rare.

Other parasitic infections such as cysticercosis (*Taenia solium*), roundworms (*Ascaris lumbricoides*) (Fig. 1.12.1) and hydatid disease (*Echinococcus granulosus*) (Fig. 1.12.2) can give characteristic radiological appearances.

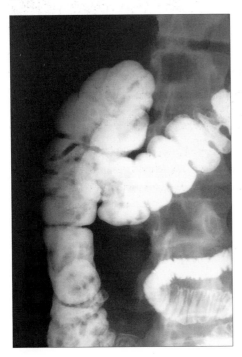

Fig. 1.12.1

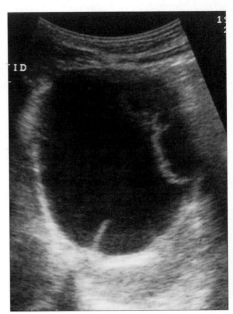

Fig. 1.12.2

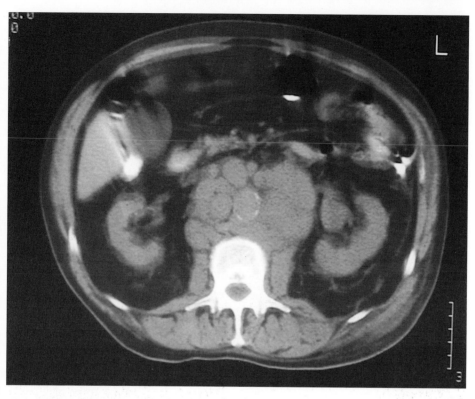

This abdominal CT scan is of a 54-year-old man with a long history of coeliac disease well controlled by diet who is being investigated for recent onset of loss of weight and increasing abdominal discomfort.

A Describe the abnormality and suggest a cause.
B Is the history of coeliac disease relevant?
C Outline treatment.

A There is gross para-aortic lympha-denopathy, which is highly suggestive of lymphoma although a similar appearance may occur in metastatic disease.

B In view of the long history of coeliac disease and symptoms the most likely diagnosis is a T-cell small bowel lymphoma.

C Surgical debulking may be required followed by chemotherapy and possibly radiotherapy depending upon the stage of the lymphoma.

Malignant tumours of the small bowel are uncommon. However, patients with coeliac disease are at a significantly higher risk; up to 10% of these patients develop T-cell lymphomas. The majority of small bowel lymphomas unrelated to coeliac disease are non-Hodgkin's B-cell lymphomas. Most tumours arise in the distal ileum, and small bowel contrast studies are useful to localize disease (Fig. 1.13.1;

distal ileal stenosis). Formal diagnosis requires biopsy whereas staging requires chest and abdominal CT scanning and bone marrow biopsy. Lymph node involvement may be relatively subtle as in Figure 1.13.2, which demonstrates involvement of the mesenteric lymph nodes.

Tumours of small bowel

- Primary
    Benign
        leiomyoma
        lipoma
        adenoma
    Malignant
        lymphoma
        carcinoid
        adenocarcinoma
        leiomyosarcoma

- Secondary
    breast/melanoma and bronchus
    adjacent abdominal malignancies
    (colon, ovary, stomach etc.)

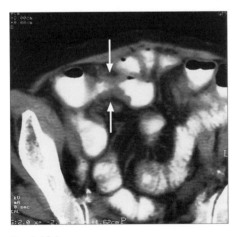

Fig. 1.13.1

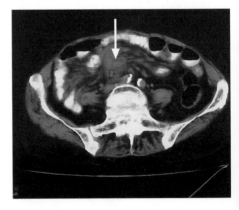

Fig. 1.13.2

QUESTION 1.14

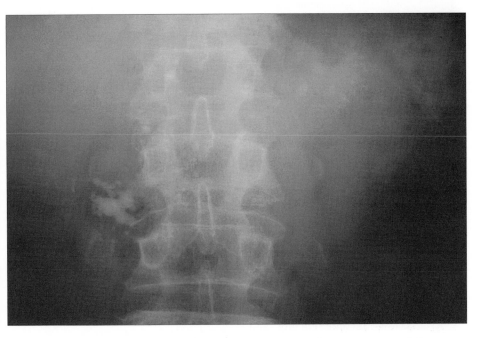

This close-up of a plain abdominal X-ray is of a 54-year-old man with intermittent severe dyspepsia.

A Describe the abnormality and suggest a diagnosis.
B What further investigations are indicated?
C What are the risk factors?
D What complications may arise and what treatment is available?

ANSWER 1.14

A There is calcification (pancreato-lithiasis) affecting primarily the head of the pancreas. This patient has chronic pancreatitis.

B If the patient has pain then an amylase test should be performed. Liver function tests may be abnormal (chole-stasis secondary to compression of common bile duct). Diabetes and glucose intolerance should be excluded. Steator-rhoea may be confirmed with a faecal fat estimation, and pancreatic exocrine insufficiency by decreased faecal chymo-trypsin levels or by response to treatment with pancreatic enzyme supplements. Note that the patient's 'dyspepsia' may also be secondary to gallstones or peptic ulcer disease.

C Risk factors include ethanol and previous recurrent episodes of acute pancreatitis.

D Complications include malabsorp-tion with resultant malnutrition, diabetes mellitus and addiction to narcotic anal-gesics. A minority of patients develop pancreatic cancer. Treatment consists of surgical correction of any remediable biliary tract disease. Alcohol intake must be discontinued and the patient should be commenced on a low-fat diet with pancreatic enzyme supplements and H_2-antagonists (reduces inactivation of enzymes). Surgical treatment may be indicated to alleviate obstruction of the pancreatic duct. Coeliac nerve blocks may be helpful for chronic pain. Subtotal or total pancreatectomy is a last resort.

A plain abdominal X-ray may prove diag-nostic in chronic pancreatitis. Pancreatic calcification occurs more commonly in chronic pancreatitis secondary to excessive alcohol ingestion than in biliary disease. Pancreatic calcification is limited to the head or tail of the pancreas in about one-quarter of cases. CT scanning is much more sensitive in the detection of calcific changes than plain film assessment (Fig. 1.14.1). ERCP may demonstrate dilated ducts, stones and strictures.

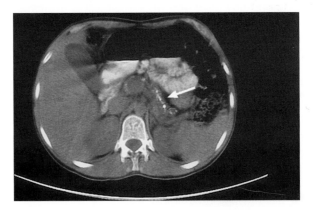

Fig. 1.14.1

QUESTION 1.15

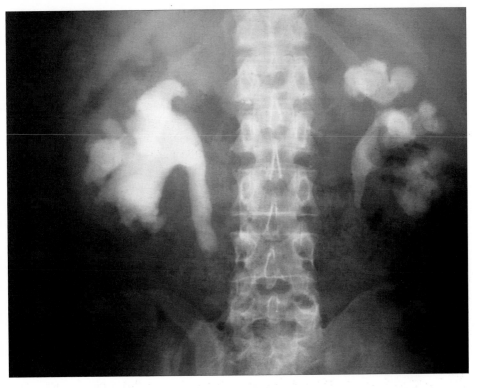

This plain abdominal X-ray is of a 44-year-old woman with a history of intermittent urinary tract infections.

A Suggest a diagnosis.
B Outline the aetiology of this disorder.
C What further investigations are indicated?
D What treatment is available?

A There are bilateral staghorn renal calculi.

B Staghorn calculi are composed of magnesium ammonium phosphate and are usually found in women with recurrent urinary sepsis with urease-producing organisms such as *Proteus*.

C An MSU is required to exclude active infection together with measurement of serum creatinine.

D Despite the large size of these calculi they can be amenable to a percutaneous nephrolithotomy (with antibiotic cover). They may recur quickly and patients should be advised to maintain a high fluid input and infection should be actively sought and treated. Fragmentation of a previously intact staghorn calculus is a useful sign of pyonephrosis.

Renal calculi may also be secondary to hypercalcaemia, hypercalciuria, hyperoxaluria, hyperuricosuria or hypocitraturia. Renal calculi may be apparent on a plain X-ray (Fig. 1.15.1, stone obstructing ureter required nephostomy). Clusters of small round calculi may be found around the apices of the renal pyramids in medullary sponge kidney (Fig. 1.15.2).

There are several important causes of renal calcification not relating to stone disease.

Commonest causes of non-stone calcification

- Infection
  TB
  Xanthogranulomatous pyelonephritis
  (hydatid)

- Carcinoma (6% of tumours calcify)

- Renal papillary necrosis

- Renal tubular acidosis

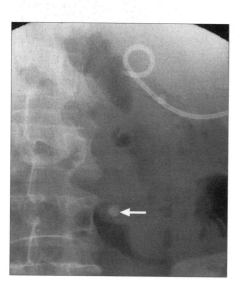

Fig. 1.15.1

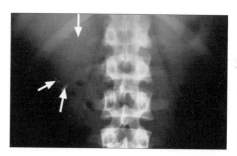

Fig. 1.15.2

QUESTION 1.16

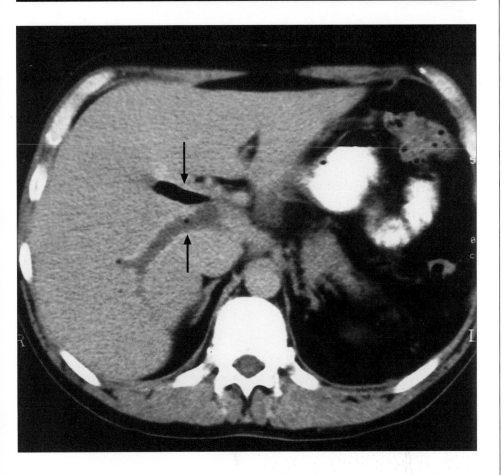

This upper abdominal CT scan (contrast-enhanced) is of a young man who had become increasingly unwell after an episode of *Salmonella typhimurium* food poisoning.

A What are the important imaging findings on this scan (arrows) and what is the clinical diagnosis?

B What are the salient clinical features of this condition?

C Outline the main areas of clinical management.

ANSWER 1.16

A There is air within the biliary tree (top arrow). The portal vein has a low density with rim-like peripheral enhancement and some additional tiny loculi of gas. This is portal vein thrombosis (bottom arrow). Additional extension of thrombus can be identified within the superior mesenteric vein (Fig. 1.16.1, arrow).

B This is an acute portal vein thrombosis with involvement of the superior mesenteric vein as a result of portal pyaemia. The acute presentation is usually with pyrexia, painful hepatomegaly, leucocytosis and possible hepatic abscess formation. Acute ascites, intestinal infarction or haemorrhage are occasionally encountered.

C Clinical management involves treating the underlying prime condition (e.g. sepsis), careful fluid balance and close clinical and biochemical monitoring. Anticoagulation and thrombolysis are also therapeutic options.

Causes of PV thrombosis

- Idiopathic (? related to previous neonatal sepsis)
- Tumour invasion (cholangiocarcinoma)
- Trauma
- Dehydration
- Sepsis (e.g. appendicitis/diverticulitis)
- Pancreatitis
- Alpha-1-antitrypsin deficiency

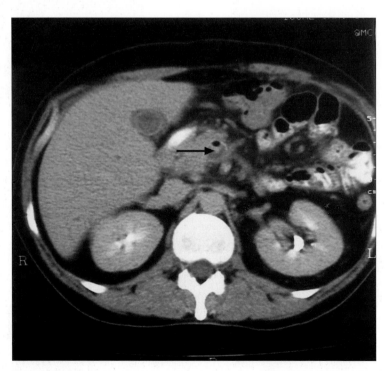

Fig. 1.16.1

BONE
RADIOLOGY

Introduction: bone radiology

Plain radiographs remain the mainstay of musculoskeletal radiology. Radio-isotope bone scans demonstrate regions of increased bone activity. The role of ultrasound and cross-sectional imaging, particularly MRI, is increasing. MRI can assess subtle bone marrow abnormalities and visualise tendons, ligaments and cartilage.

For examination purposes candidates should be familiar with the plain radiographic skeletal manifestations of several medical conditions, including arthritides, metabolic bone disease, haematological disorders and miscellaneous conditions such as Paget's disease.

When examining a musculoskeletal radiograph one should assess the following.

Appearance of the bones

- Epiphyseal maturity: retarded, generalised or localised. Fragmentation: avascular necrosis.
- Presence of transverse lines of increased density. This occurs in hypervitaminosis D, scurvy, leukaemia and lead poisoning.
- Integrity of cortical margins and presence of periosteal reaction. New bone formation from osteoblasts may raise periosteum which can be diffuse or localised.
- Density. Look for generalised/localised osteoporosis (diminished calcium content due to diminution of protein bone matrix), osteomalacia (deficient mineralisation of bone due to lack of calcium or vitamin D), localised translucent (osteolytic) region which may be well or poorly circumscribed, mixed osteolytic and osteosclerotic lesions. The main distinction in this appearance is between infective and neoplastic lesions: histological confirmation is often required.
- Presence of dysplasia. Check if epiphyseal, physeal, metaphyseal and diaphyseal; generalised/localised.

Joint abnormalities

- Single/multiple. Monoarticular involvement is usually due to a localised process – post-traumatic, infectious or degenerative. Polyarticular disorders are seen with systemic diseases such as rheumatoid arthritis (RA) and psoriatic arthropathy.
- Symmetry. RA is typically bilaterally symmetrical; degenerative joint disease (DJD) is usually unilateral/bilaterally asymmetrical.
- Distribution of joints involved. Some arthritides tend to involve peripheral joints (hands and feet) more prominently (RA and gout); anklyosing spondylitis affects the proximal large joints and spine.
- Joint space. This reflects presence or absence of additional fluid and the condition of articular cartilage.
- Inflammatory arthropathies (RA) result in uniform loss of joint space. In DJD, joint space narrowing is more localised/uneven.
- Erosions imply an inflammatory pathology.
- Alignment of bones at joints. Deviation may occur, e.g. ulnar at metacarpophalangeal.

Appearance of soft tissues

- Localised/generalised increase or decrease in prominence.
- Presence of calcification in cartilage or surrounding soft tissues.

With regard to skull radiographs see Section 4.

QUESTION 2.1

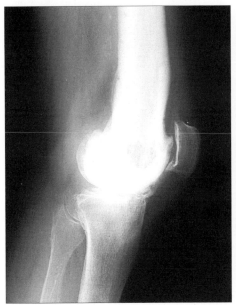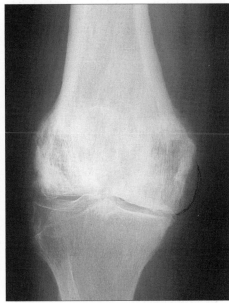

This knee X-ray is of a 74-year-old woman who complains of intermittent knee pain.

A Describe the abnormality.
B What condition does this patient have and what physical sign may be present?
C What complications may arise?
D What treatment is available and how may it be monitored?

ANSWER 2.1

A The distal femur is expanded and demonstrates abnormal coarsened bone texture and sclerosis.

B Paget's disease. A soft bruit may be audible secondary to the increased blood flow through the pagetic bone. When bones such as the tibia are affected the overlying soft tissues may be warm to the touch.

C Pathological fractures may occur and usually affect weight-bearing bones such as the femur. Secondary osteoarthritis may be troublesome, whereas high-output congestive cardiac failure and malignant change are uncommon. Patients may develop nerve compression syndromes that may affect cranial nerves (usually I, II or VIII) or nerve roots. Platybasia with basilar invagination may cause hydrocephalus or brainstem compression.

D Treatment is indicated to alleviate symptoms and prevent or treat complications. Analgesics and anti-inflammatory drugs may be sufficient for minor discomfort or secondary arthritic changes whereas biphosphonates or calcitonin may be indicated for more severe disease. Mithramycin is used less commonly in view of its bone marrow toxicity. Orthopaedic surgery, including joint replacement, may be considered although it is usually preceded by medical treatment to reduce bone vascularity. Treatment is usually monitored by following the level of serum bony alkaline phosphatase although urinary hydroxyproline can also be used. X-ray appearance is also useful.

Paget's disease may affect any bone but the most commonly affected is the pelvis (76%); other common sites include the dorsal (20%) and lumbar (33%) spine, the sacrum (28%), the skull (28%) and the femur (25%). The hands and feet are not usually involved. Paget's disease may be monostotic or polyostotic and typically produces an enlarged, expanded appearance with cortical thickening and coarse trabecular markings with lytic or sclerotic changes. It is characterized by an initial destructive phase which is followed by the reparative phase during which there may be a mixed sclerotic and lytic pattern to the bone. In the later sclerotic phase the disease may simulate osteoblastic metastases such as occur in prostatic or breast carcinoma (Fig. 2.1.1, metastatic disease).

Skull X-ray appearances include osteoporosis circumscripta (early destructive phase with sharply demarcated radioluscent area), which progresses to the more mottled 'cotton wool' appearance as areas of sclerosis develop (Fig. 2.1.2).

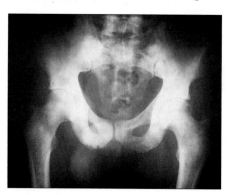

Fig. 2.1.1

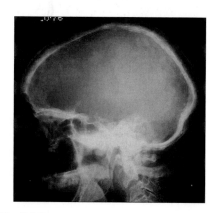

Fig. 2.1.2

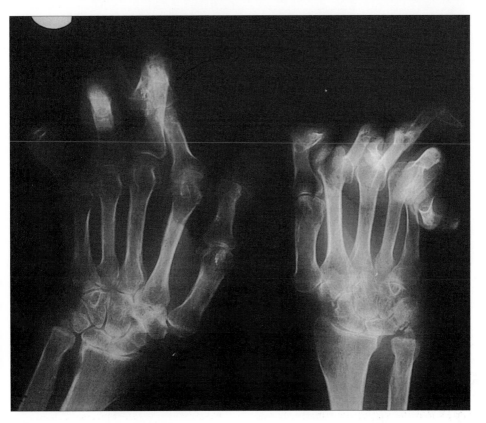

This X-ray is of a 54-year-old man from Thailand who has palpable peripheral nerves.

A Describe the abnormality and suggest a diagnosis.
B How is the diagnosis made and what other clinical signs may be present?
C What treatment is available?
D Suggest two other possible diagnoses that may give an identical radiological appearance.

A There is a severe mutilating arthropathy with gross destruction of the terminal tufts of the phalanges together with arthritic changes affecting the carpus and other small joints. In view of the palpable nerves the most likely diagnosis is leprosy (Hansen's disease).

B The diagnosis is usually made clinically although confirmatory skin biopsies and slit skin smears are helpful. Clinical signs include a severe distal sensory neuropathy, anaesthetic skin lesions and trophic ulceration and scarring. Patients classically have thickened peripheral nerves (e.g. posterior tibial, ulnar and greater auricular nerves) as well as alopecia.

C Treatment includes various combinations of dapsone (screen for glucose-6-phosphate dehydrogenase deficiency before treatment), rifampicin and clofazimine. Prednisolone may need to be added if reactions to drug treatment occur.

D This radiological appearance may be found in other severe neuropathic conditions such as syringomyelia, tabes dorsalis or longstanding severe diabetes mellitus.

There are a variety of conditions that can result in marked erosion of the terminal phalangeal tufts. The arthritis mutilans variety of psoriatic arthropathy can produce severe phalangeal 'whittling' together with irregular bony destruction. The repeated self-injury inflicted by patients with the Lesch–Nyhan syndrome can produce a similar appearance. Terminal phalangeal resorption may also occur in scleroderma together with epidermolysis bullosa and conditions associated with severe vascular ischaemia such as diabetes mellitus and thromboangiitis obliterans. Severe neuropathies may lead to the development of Charcot joints, which should suggest longstanding diabetes mellitus (Fig. 2.2.1), or treponemal disease if in the lower limb and leprosy or syringomyelia (Fig. 2.2.2) if affecting the upper limb.

Causes of acro-osteolysis (erosion of terminal phalangeal tufts)

- Psoriatic arthropathy
- Neuropathic arthropathy
- Hyperparathyroidism
- Scleroderma
- Epidermolysis bullosa

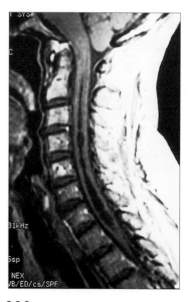

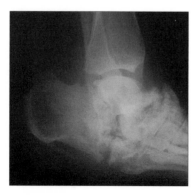

Fig. 2.2.1

Fig. 2.2.2

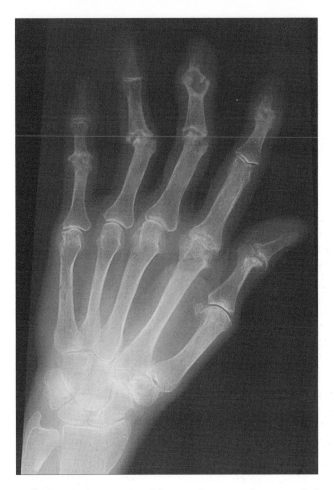

This X-ray is from a 66-year-old renal transplant recipient who suffers with intermittent joint pains.

A Describe the abnormality.
B Suggest a diagnosis and further investigation.
C What treatment may be offered?

ANSWER 2.3

A There are arthritic changes affecting the carpus and the metacarpophalangeal and interphalangeal joints. However, the most marked abnormality is a large punched-out erosion affecting the middle finger distal interphalangeal joint.

B This appearance suggests a gouty arthropathy. A serum uric acid level is required.

C Treatment is indicated for gouty arthropathy, gouty nephropathy or for recurrent episodes of pain. Allopurinol (± prophylactic colchicine or NSAIDs) is used more commonly than uricosuric agents such as probenecid or sulphinpyrazone. NSAIDs should be avoided in renal transplant recipients. In addition, allopurinol markedly potentiates the action of azathioprine and should be avoided completely or used in a very small dose with strict monitoring of the white cell count. Acute episodes of gout in this patient may be treated by a course of colchicine or an increased dose of prednisolone.

Longstanding gout results in the formation of tophi, which may be evident on bone X-rays as soft-tissue swelling. A characteristic feature is the 'rat bite' erosion (Fig. 2.3.1), which may be large with a well defined margin. As the erosion enlarges it usually involves more of the shaft than the articular surface. Gout tends mainly to involve the distal and proximal interphalangeal joints. Severe destruction can occur in advanced disease. Subcutaneous calcification may be found in scleroderma (Fig. 2.3.2, little finger), Raynaud's phenomenon, dermatomyositis, polymyositis, gout or hyperparathyroidism. Osteoarthritis typically affects the distal interphalangeal joints and thumb carpometacarpal joints (Fig. 2.3.3).

Common causes of gout

- Primary
- Secondary: myeolproliferative disorders, endocrine (hyperparathyroidism and myxoedema), chronic renal failure

---

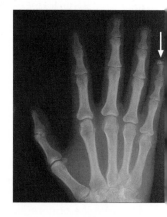

Fig. 2.3.2

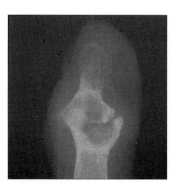

Fig. 2.3.1

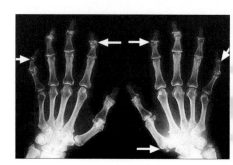

Fig. 2.3.3

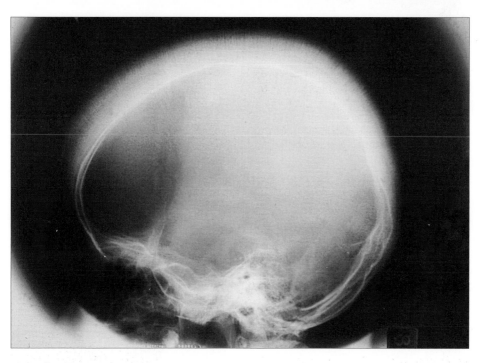

This skull X-ray is of a 24-year-old woman.

A Describe the abnormality and suggest an underlying diagnosis.

ANSWER 2.4

A The skull is markedly abnormal with gross thickening of the skull vault, which has a 'hair-on-end' appearance. This suggests a diagnosis of a severe congenital haemolytic anaemia.

Such conditions result in hyperplastic bone marrow, which causes expansion of the diploic space with subsequent thinning of the outer table of the skull. Note that the inferior occipital bone is not involved as it contains little bone marrow. Other features include poor development of the sinuses and forward displacement of the upper central incisors, producing dental malocclusion. Other characteristic skull X-ray appearances include the 'copper beaten' appearance of chronic raised intracranial pressure (Fig. 2.4.1) and the, albeit more subtle, diffuse pattern of skull demineralization seen in hyperparathyroidism (Fig. 2.4.2). Chronic raised intracranial pressure also leads to the erosion of the dorsum sellae.

Causes of 'hair-on-end' appearance

- Haemolytic anaemias
  - thalassaemia major
  - hereditary spherocytosis
  - sickle cell disease
- Congenital cyanotic heart disease

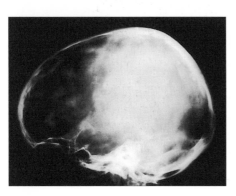

Fig. 2.4.1

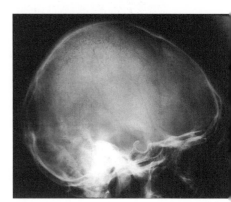

Fig. 2.4.2

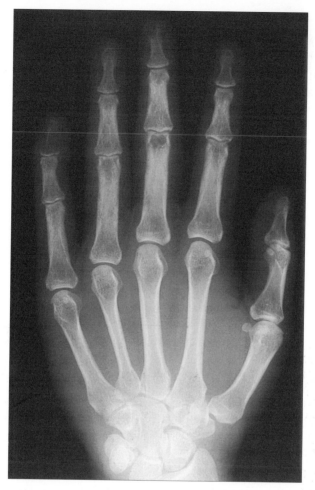

This hand X-ray is of a 25-year-old man who is on renal replacement therapy.

A Describe the abnormality and suggest a diagnosis.
B Explain the pathogenesis.
C What treatment is available?

ANSWER 2.5

A There is subperiosteal resorption of the phalanges evident secondary to tertiary hyperparathyroidism.

B Renal failure is accompanied by hyperphosphataemia, hypocalcaemia and markedly lowered levels of 1,25-dihydroxycholecalciferol. These factors result in a stimulation of PTH secretion (secondary hyperparathyroidism), which initially leads to correction of the hypocalcaemia; however, this is at the expense of bone integrity such that patients develop osteitis fibrosa cystica. Bone disease worsens when autonomous tertiary hyperparathyroidism develops.

C Initial treatment consists of reducing phosphate levels with a combination of dietary restriction and calcium-containing phosphate binders. A vitamin D analogue is then added to increase intestinal calcium absorption and directly inhibit PTH secretion. However, patients with advanced bone disease usually require a surgical parathyroidectomy and long-term treatment with calcitriol or a similar agent.

The subperiosteal erosions of hyperparathyroidism typically affect the radial side of the phalanx and in severe disease the terminal phalanx may be significantly eroded (Fig. 2.5.1). Brown tumours may develop (Fig. 2.5.2 – expanded lytic rib lesion). Brown tumours are actually cysts resulting from intraosseous haemorrhage. They are generally well demarcated, cause bony expansion and can be a site of pathological fracture.

Skeletal signs of hyper-PTH

- Subperiosteal bone resorption
- Cortical tunnelling ('pepper pot skull')
- Bone softening – basilar invagination and pathological fractures
- Brown tumours
- Soft-tissue calcification
- Marginal erosion of joints and acro-osteolysis
- Chondrocalcinosis

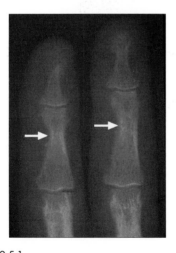

Fig. 2.5.1

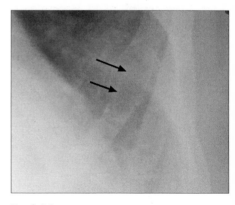

Fig. 2.5.2

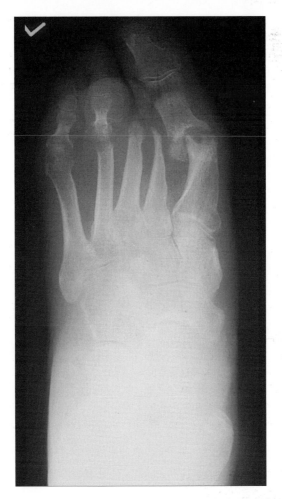

This X-ray is of a 42-year-old man who was admitted to hospital in septicaemic shock.

A   Describe the abnormality and suggest a diagnosis and an underlying cause.
B   What treatment is required?

ANSWER 2.6

A There is marked destruction of the first metatarsophalangeal joint with loss of the second and third toes. The septicaemic illness is probably secondary to chronic osteomyelitis in a patient with longstanding diabetes mellitus.

B This patient requires intravenous antibiotics, tight glycaemic control and adequate treatment of the osteomyelitis, which may include a surgical debridement together with a prolonged course of antibiotics.

The 'diabetic foot' is particularly prone to develop osteomyelitis as a consequence of the development of neuropathic ulcers that act as a source of infection. Treatment consists of surgical debridement, which may need to be extensive (Fig. 2.6.1) in order to remove all the infected material, combined with antibiotic therapy. From the MRCP point of view osteomyelitis on a foot X-ray with evidence of either previous amputation or marked vascular calcification is secondary to diabetes mellitus.

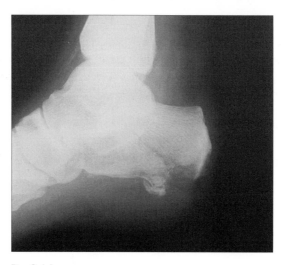

Fig. 2.6.1

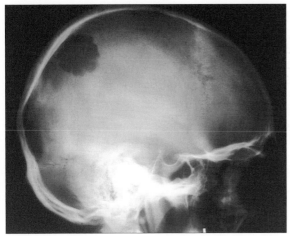

A

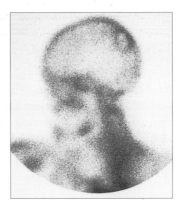

B

Film A is a skull X-ray whereas film B is an isotope scan of a 22-year-old man who has a history of a nonproductive cough, exertional dyspnoea, occasional fever, mild weight loss, polydipsia and polyuria.

A Describe the abnormality and suggest a diagnosis.
B What complications may arise?
C What treatment is available?

A There is a well demarcated lytic lesion in the vault of the skull. This is very unlikely to be a metastatic or infective lesion as there is no increased uptake on the isotope scan. This radiological appearance in a young adult with a history suggesting a systemic disorder with pulmonary involvement and polyuria/polydipsia strongly suggests Langerhans' cell histiocytosis (previously called Histiocytosis X). This lesion is therefore an eosinophilic granuloma.

B Complications include progressive lung disease, recurrent pneumothoraces, pathological fractures secondary to cystic bone lesions and diabetes insipidus.

C The disease is associated with and exacerbated by smoking. Abstinence is therefore an important aspect of treatment. Corticosteroids and cytotoxic drugs have been used in this disease but their exact role is still not clear.

Langerhans' cell histiocytosis is an uncommon disease and typically affects young adults. The lesions are characterized histologically by the presence of eosinophilic histiocytes. The lung involvement predominantly affects the mid and upper zones (Fig. 2.7.1), in contrast to fibrosing alveolitis. Appearances include reticulonodular infiltrates and cystic or ill-defined nodular lesions. Progressive disease may lead to marked fibrosis and honeycombing. The sparing of the costophrenic angles is a characteristic feature of pulmonary disease and is a good prognostic indicator as its absence is associated with progressive disease.

Most affected patients have asymptomatic bony involvement, with a minority having the multiple system manifestations.

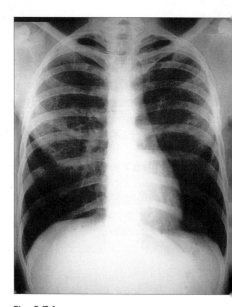

Fig. 2.7.1

QUESTION 2.8

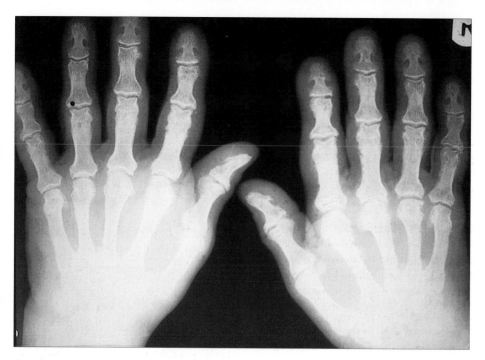

This hand X-ray is of a 55-year-old man with hypertension.

A Describe the abnormality and suggest a diagnosis.
B What further investigations are indicated?
C What complications may arise?
D What treatment is available?

A The hand is broad and spade-like with marked broadening of the distal phalangeal tufts (Fig. 2.8.1). This patient has acromegaly.

B The diagnosis may be confirmed by a failure of suppression of growth hormone (GH) levels in response to oral glucose. Fasting levels of insulin-like growth factor 1 (IGF-1) are usually markedly elevated and can be used to monitor treatment. Fasting serum prolactin may be elevated as it is often also secreted by GH-secreting tumours. A fasting glucose test, thyroid function tests and routine haematology and biochemistry is indicated. Imaging of the pituitary fossa reveals an adenoma in about 90% of patients (Fig. 2.8.2).

C Patients may have a typical appearance (prognathism, dental malocclusion, oily sweaty skin, with large doughy extremities). Complications are myriad and include hypertension, diabetes mellitus, hypopituitarism (particularly secondary hypothyroidism and hypogonadism), cardiac hypertrophy, cardiac failure, carpal tunnel syndrome, chondrocalcinosis and arthritis, bitemporal hemianopia (caused by optic chiasma pressure – Fig. 2.8.3) and spinal cord compression.

D Treatment may be surgical (transsphenoidal hypophysectomy), local radiation therapy or medical such as bromocriptine or octreotide.

Other features of acromegaly that may be apparent on X-rays include an enlarged pituitary fossa and frontal sinuses with thickening of the skull vault, cardiac hypertrophy, thickening of the heel pad, chondrocalcinosis and secondary arthritis.

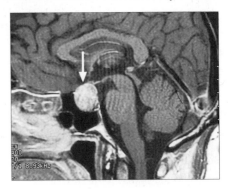

Fig. 2.8.2

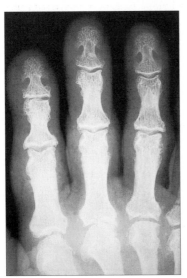

Fig. 2.8.1

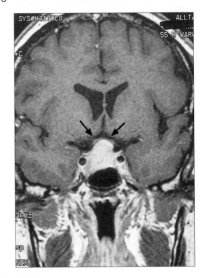

Fig. 2.8.3

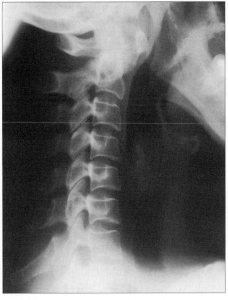

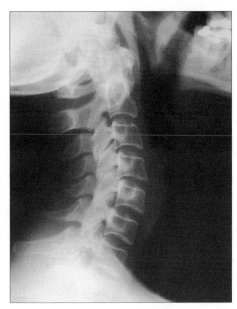

A   **B**

Films A and B are flexion and extension cervical spine X-rays of a 44-year-old woman who complains of increasing muscular weakness and urinary difficulties.

A Describe the abnormality and suggest a diagnosis.
B What treatment is required?
C What clinical signs would suggest multiple sclerosis as a potential cause of her symptoms?

A There is marked anterior sub-luxation of the atlas with respect to the odontoid peg. Atlantoaxial subluxation may be secondary to trauma but is more commonly associated with rheumatoid arthritis and does not correlate with the severity of the arthritis. This patient has clinical symptoms of spinal cord compression.

B Treatment may be conservative with a cervical collar or other forms of cervical brace, but surgical fixation may be indi-cated depending on the degree of spinal cord compression.

C The presence of optic atrophy, a brisk jaw jerk or dysarthria would sug-gest a disease process above and below the level of the foramen magnum, as seen in demyelination.

Patients with atlantoaxial subluxation often require further imaging with a CT or MRI scan (Fig. 2.9.1) to determine whether the degree of spinal cord involvement is severe. Rheumatoid arthritis is an erosive arthropathy and may involve many joints, including shoulder joints (Fig. 2.9.2, note pulmonary fibrosis), knees, feet and hands (Fig. 2.9.3, multiple surgical procedures are evident).

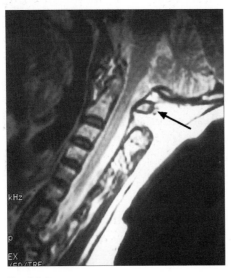

Fig. 2.9.1

> **Plain film signs of rheumatoid arthritis**
>
> - Widened joint space and soft-tissue swel-ling (effusion and synovial inflammation)
> - Ostepaenia (hyperaemia and disuse)
> - Joint space narrowing (cartilage destruc-tion by pannus)
> - Periarticular erosions (destruction of bone by pannus)
> - Ligament and capsular laxity – sub-luxation and deformity
> - Fibrosis and ankylosis (cartilaginous joints are less severely involved)

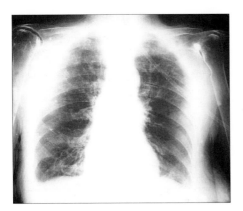

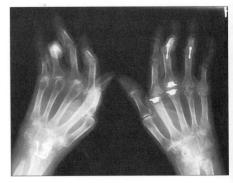

Fig. 2.9.2   Fig. 2.9.3

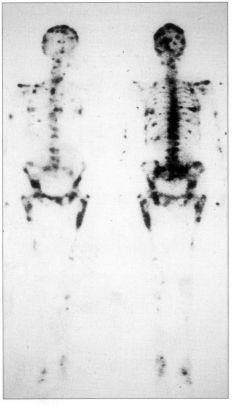

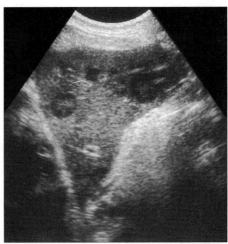

A   **B**

Film A is an isotope bone scan and film B a hepatic ultrasound scan of a nonsmoking 66-year-old woman who gives a history of anorexia, weakness and worsening arthritis.

A Describe the abnormalities and suggest an underlying diagnosis.
B What treatment is available?

A The bone scan demonstrates multiple areas of increased uptake ('hot spots') throughout the skeleton although multiple hypoechoic lesions are evident on the liver ultrasound. This patient has disseminated malignancy. In a woman of this age the most likely diagnosis is carcinoma of the breast.

B At this advanced stage treatment is palliative. Radiotherapy is useful for bone pain, preventing pathological fractures and local disease such as tumour ulceration or soft-tissue metastases. Hormonal manipulation with tamoxifen may be of benefit in pre- and postmenopausal women. Patients may respond to combination chemotherapy with cytotoxic drugs such as doxorubicin, cyclophosphamide and vincristine. Recently there has been increasing interest in the use of high-dose ablative chemotherapy in combination with autologous bone marrow or stem cell transplant in patients with metastatic breast cancer, but hard data is currently lacking.

Bone scans play an important role in the assessment of metastatic disease. However, increased uptake of isotope is also seen in conditions such as Paget's disease (Fig. 2.10.1) and hyperparathyroidism where there is increased bone turnover producing the so-called 'super scan' appearance with a uniform marked increase in uptake in the axial skeleton (Fig. 2.10.2).

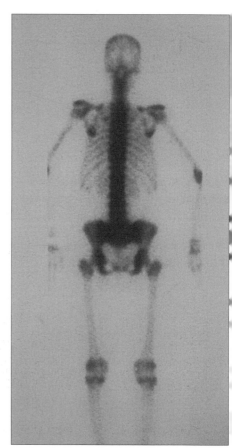

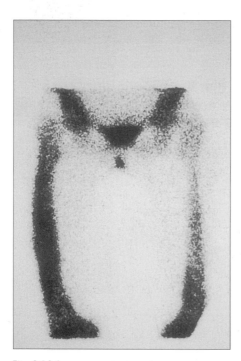

Fig. 2.10.1

Fig. 2.10.2

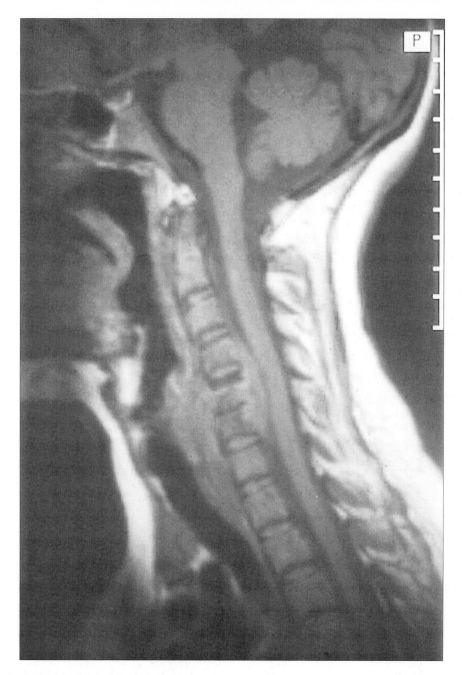

This MRI scan of the cervical spine is of a 31-year-old Asian woman who gives a history of lethargy and general malaise.

A Describe the abnormality and suggest an underlying diagnosis.
B Outline treatment.

A This is a T1-w scan as the CSF has a low signal (dark). At the C4–6 levels there is a soft-tissue mass extending anteriorly into the prevertebral soft tissues and posteriorly, and compressing the spinal theca. There is some vertebral body destruction (especially C5). These appearances are of a vertebral abscess in the lower cervical region. The differential diagnosis includes a pyogenic or tuberculous abscess; the latter is more common in Asian patients.

B A definitive diagnosis is required therefore aspiration and biopsy of the lesion is indicated. Broad spectrum intravenous antibiotics or combination chemotherapy is required in the case of a pyogenic or tuberculous abscess, respectively.

MRI scans are extremely useful in the investigation of disease involving the spine and paravertebral tissues. Lesions easily detectable include external spinal cord compression from degenerative disease of the cervical vertebrae (Fig. 2.11.1, cervical myelopathy), herniation of intervertebral discs (Fig. 2.11.2) or extramedullary primary or metastatic tumours. Intramedullary lesions such as demyelination, neurosarcoidosis, syringomyelia or primary tumours are also readily identifiable.

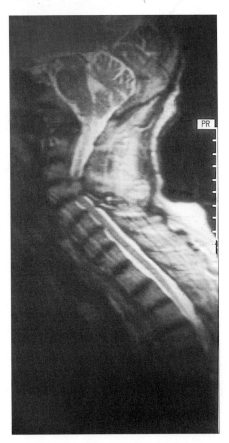

Fig. 2.11.1

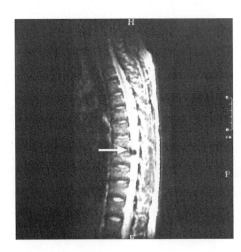

Fig. 2.11.2

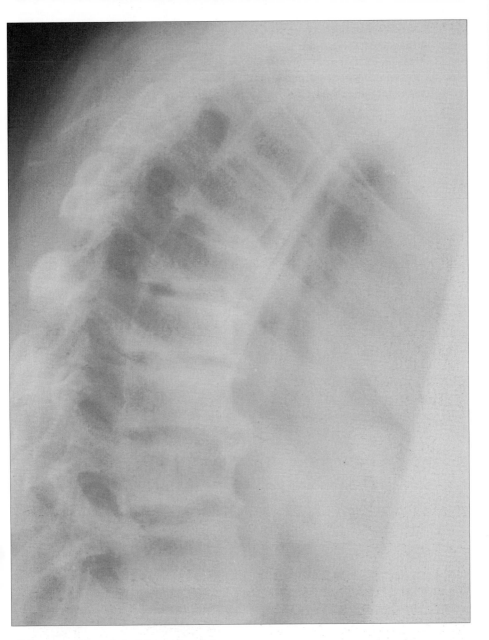

This X-ray is of a 52-year-old man.

A Describe the abnormality and suggest a diagnosis.

A The vertebrae have the classic 'rugger jersey' appearance (horizontal sclerotic bands adjacent to vertebral body end-plates) of renal osteodystrophy. This patient has renal bone disease.

Imaging of the spine may exhibit changes secondary to degenerative, metabolic, neoplastic or infective disease processes. Examples include partial or complete vertebral collapse in osteoporosis (Fig. 2.12.1), vertebral collapse secondary to malignant infiltration (Fig. 2.12.2 – myeloma), Gibbus formation after spinal tuberculosis (Fig. 2.12.3). This MRI scan is T2-w as the CSF has a high signal (appears white).

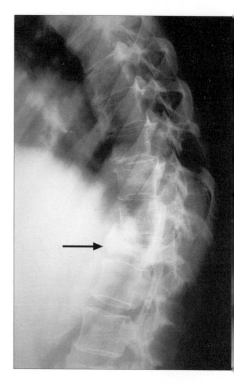

Fig. 2.12.2

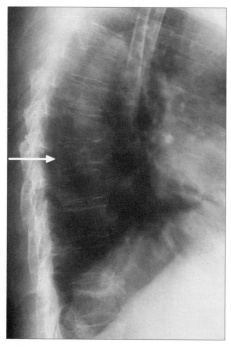

Fig. 2.12.1

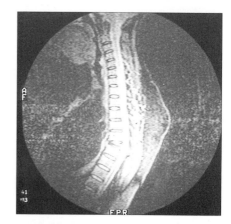

Fig. 2.12.3

CONTRAST IMAGES

Introduction: contrast images

Image interpretation is based on being able to discern between one structure and another. When their relative appearance/natural contrast (attenuation) is similar, addition of a contrast agent to one structure can make it stand out. X-ray contrast enhancing agents (iodine and barium) act by increasing the local absorption of X-rays wherever they are distributed. Contrast may be used to delineate the arterial and venous systems. During fluoroscopic studies, body cavities and viscera can be outlined. The genitourinary tract may also be imaged by the administration of intravenous contrast media because of the preferred route of renal excretion — the intravenous urogram (IVU). Filling defects, strictures and sites of obstruction may be demonstrated.

Studies of the vascular tree and IVUs utilise iodine-based contrast media. As with all drugs, contrast media may invoke an anaphylactic response. There is a lower incidence of adverse reaction with the newer low-osmolar agents. Nephrotoxicity has an incidence of up to 5%. For the majority, renal impairment is temporary. Predisposing factors include pre-existing impaired renal function, diabetes mellitus, dehydration and multiple myeloma.

There are two major types of contrast agents used to image the bowel during fluoroscopic studies: barium and water-soluble iodinated contrast, such as gastrograffin. Barium, being denser, is utilised in double contrast studies in which the organ is distended with gas (or air) and the mucosa is coated with contrast media. Water-soluble contrast media may be utilised for single contrast studies in situations in which barium is contraindicated, such as suspected perforation. In CT imaging the concentration of contrast for bowel opacification is comparatively very low, as the preparations used for conventional radiography produce severe artefact on CT. Standard barium studies should be avoided in patients in whom CT is planned within the next few days.

The natural contrast within an organ during CT may be made more prominent by administering intravenous contrast media, a process referred to as 'enhancement'. In MRI, gadolinium DTPA, a paramagnetic agent, changes the local magnetic environment of the tissue in which it is distributed thereby influencing the MR relaxation rates. The presence of a contrast agent in and around an abnormality may aid the characterisation of a lesion. Cross-sectional imaging of all body regions frequently encompasses contrast enhanced studies.

As with all imaging, studying the film beyond the region outlined by contrast for other findings is recommended to note incidental pathology or an alternative cause for the symptoms other than that which the current investigation is assessing. When available the pre-contrast or 'control' film should be studied, as the contrast may obscure relevant findings, particularly calcified structures.

Some of the questions in the other sections of this book could also be placed in this section, reflecting the widespread utilisation of contrast studies. Most of the cases in this section relate to the gastrointestinal tract topics with which the examination candidate should be familiar.

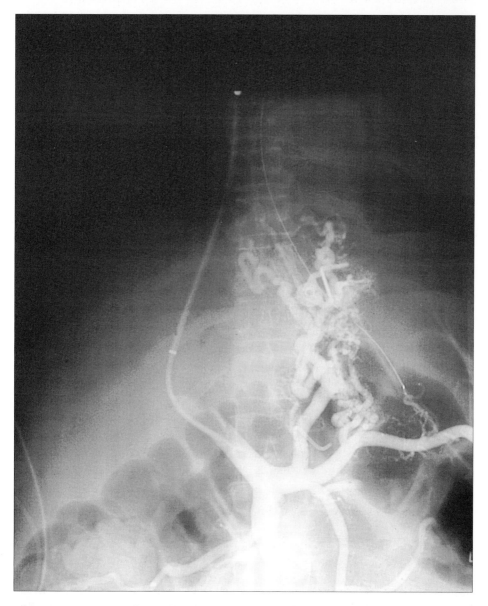

This X-ray was taken during a radiological procedure.

A What is the procedure called?
B Suggest an underlying diagnosis.
C What is the aim of this procedure?

A This procedure is called a transjugular intrahepatic portosystemic shunt (TIPS). A catheter is wedged into a tributary of the hepatic vein that communicates with the portal circulation via the liver parenchyma. The portal vein is then identified and punctured under ultrasound guidance. This tract is dilated with a balloon catheter and a self-expanding metallic stent can be inserted.

B The patient has gastro-oesophageal varices secondary to portal hypertension, which is usually the result of cirrhosis. Possible underlying aetiologies include viral hepatitis (B and C), ethanol, metabolic disorders (e.g. Wilson's disease and haemochromatosis), autoimmune disorders (e.g. primary biliary cirrhosis and autoimmune hepatitis), alpha-1-antitrypsin deficiency and drugs, although some cases are idiopathic.

C The aim is to provide a portosystemic shunt in order to decrease the pressure in the portal venous circulation.

TIPS may be used to treat acute or recurrent variceal bleeding. Elective embolization can be performed (Fig. 3.1.1). It is also useful when refractory bleeding is caused by endoscopically inaccessible intestinal or gastric varices (10–15% of patients). It may also be of use in patients with intractable ascites. Although stent placement is over 90% successful, such interventional procedures are not without complications, for example haemorrhage, sepsis, DIC and stent stenosis or occlusion. Rebleeding occurs in approximately 15% of patients. Stent closure secondary to thrombosis may be treated by low-dose thrombolysis, dilatation of the stent or stent replacement. Hepatic encephalopathy can develop in 5–35% of patients and is related to the age of the patient, the diameter of the stent and the presence of advanced liver disease. Polycystic liver disease is an absolute contraindication (distorted anatomy). Other treatments include endoscopic sclerotherapy, variceal banding, intravenous octreotide (or somatostatin or vasopressin) or insertion of a Sengstaken–Blakemore tube. Long-term treatment includes repeated endoscopic sclerotherapy/banding, beta blockers, a surgical distal splenorenal shunt or liver transplantation. Oesophageal varices may be detected incidentally by barium swallow (Fig. 3.1.2).

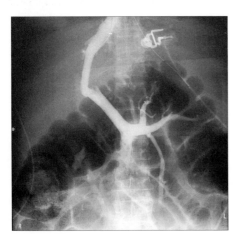

Fig. 3.1.1

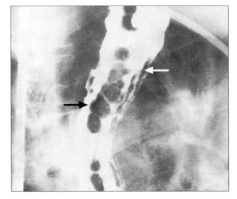

Fig. 3.1.2

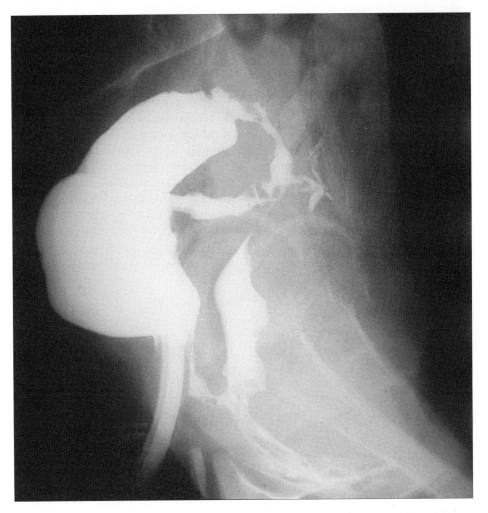

This is the barium enema of a 46-year-old woman.

A Describe the abnormality.
B Suggest a differential diagnosis.
C What treatment is available?

ANSWER 3.2

A There is a stricture of the distal colon with a fistula between the colon and the vagina such that contrast is seen spilling out onto the perineum.

B The differential diagnosis lies between Crohn's disease, diverticulitis and malignancy such as carcinoma of the cervix or colon.

C Surgical intervention is required together with therapy for the underlying condition.

Fistulae may result from inflammatory or neoplastic disease. Typical fistulating inflammatory conditions include diverticulitis and Crohn's disease; the latter often causes multiple fistulae (Fig. 3.2.1). Ulcerative colitis may lead to colonic perforation but does not usually result in fistula formation. Carcinoma of the colon, cervix or even bladder may result in fistulae.

Previous pelvic radiotherapy treatment increases the risk of fistulae, often many years after treatment. Penetrating injury and a complication of surgery account for a small proportion of the cases.

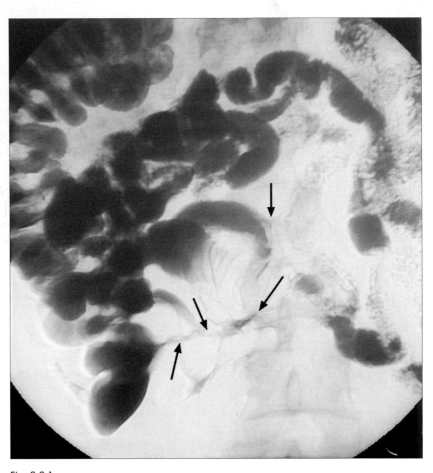

Fig. 3.2.1

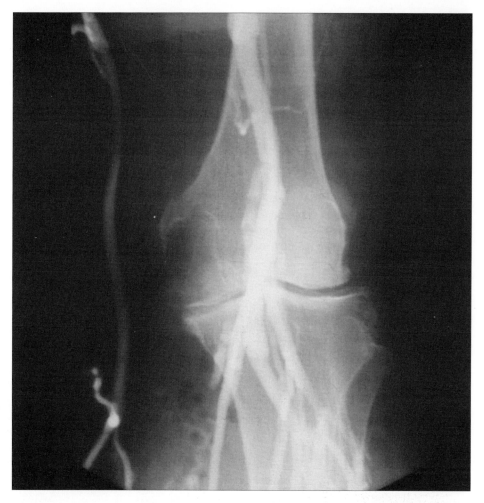

This venogram is of a 54-year-old woman with longstanding poorly controlled insulin-dependent diabetes mellitus who attended the Accident and Emergency department with a 2-day history of a painful left calf.

A Describe the abnormality.
B Suggest a diagnosis.
C What treatment is indicated?

A There is free flow of contrast with no evidence of a deep venous thrombosis. There are, however, loculi of gas within the soft tissues of the upper calf and popliteal region.

B Infection of the soft tissues with a gas-forming organism.

C Treatment includes broad spectrum intravenous antibiotics, tight glycaemic control and surgical drainage of any developing collections of pus may well be necessary. If there is any clinical evidence of a significant compartment syndrome in the lower limb, fasciotomy must be performed.

A venous thrombosis is evident as a filling defect within the lumen of a deep vein (Fig. 3.3.1). The entire deep venous system may be thrombosed and this results in filling of only the superficial veins (Fig. 3.3.2). Free gas in the soft tissues is an important radiological sign and should never be ignored. It indicates infection with gas-forming organisms that requires prompt and aggressive treatment.

Serum D-dimer levels and colour Doppler ultrasound have effectively replaced venography in the diagnosis and assessment of suspected DVT in many centres.

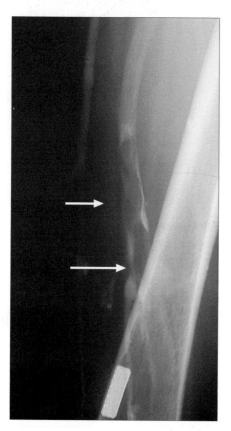

Fig. 3.3.1

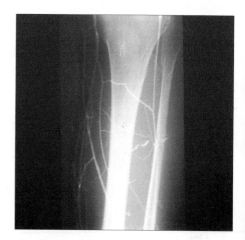

Fig. 3.3.2

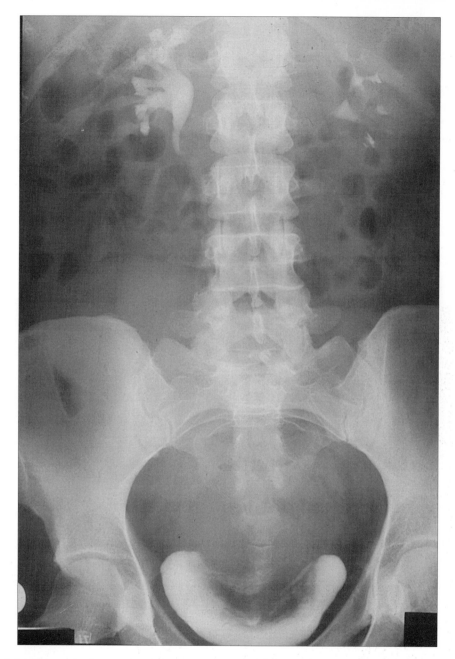

This X-ray is from an intravenous urogram of a 34-year-old woman.

A Describe the abnormalities and suggest a diagnosis.
B What further investigations are required?

ANSWER 3.4

A The left kidney is normal whereas the right kidney exhibits calyceal clubbing indicative of chronic pyelonephritis. There is a large rounded mass in the pelvis, indenting the bladder. This is unlikely to represent a normal uterus and additional pathology should be considered.

B This patient requires a pelvic ultrasound or CT scan to delineate the origin and nature of the pelvic mass.

Chronic pyelonephritis is a late sequelae of vesico-ureteric reflux (Fig. 3.4.1, micturating cystourethrogram exhibiting vesicouretic reflex or micturation) in childhood. Renal scarring results from the reflux of infected urine. Chronic pyelonephritis may be focal, diffuse, unilateral or bilateral. The affected kidney is usually smaller with clubbed, dilated calyces and cortical scarring.

Any suggestion of a pelvic mass requires further investigation. In this case CT scanning revealed bilateral ovarian cystic lesions (Fig. 3.4.2).

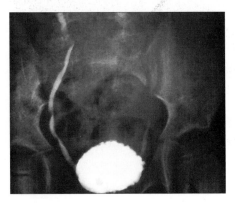

Fig. 3.4.1

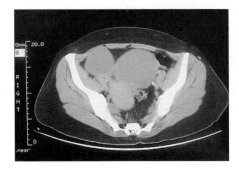

Fig. 3.4.2

QUESTION 3.5

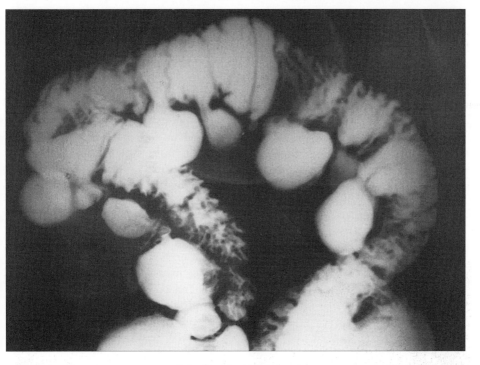

This X-ray is from a small bowel enema of a 29-year-old man who complains of loss of weight, persistent diarrhoea and general lethargy.

A Describe the abnormality and suggest a diagnosis.
B Suggest a cause for his lethargy and the further investigations that are required.
C What treatment is available?

ANSWER 3.5

A There are numerous jejunal diverticulae present, arising from the antimesenteric border. The diarrhoea is probably secondary to bacterial overgrowth.

B This patient may well have a macrocytic anaemia secondary to defective vitamin B12 and folate absorption. Further investigations required include a full blood count, blood film and measurement of folate and vitamin B12 levels (± Schilling test). Other relevant tests include the determination of faecal fat excretion to document steatorrhoea and a hydrogen breath test. Aspiration and culture of upper jejunal contents usually reveals a mixed flora with predominant *E. coli* or bacteroides.

C Surgery may be required for acute complications such as severe bleeding, diverticulitis, volvulus and perforation. An associated motility disorder such as scleroderma should be seriously considered in such patients. Patients may benefit from intermittent courses of antibiotics to limit bacterial proliferation together with fat-soluble vitamin supplementation.

Radiological investigations may be very useful in the work-up of patients with malabsorption syndromes. A small bowel enema may reveal diverticulae, fistulae and blind loops although it may only show nonspecific small bowel dilatation and thickening of the mucosal folds (Fig. 3.5.1).

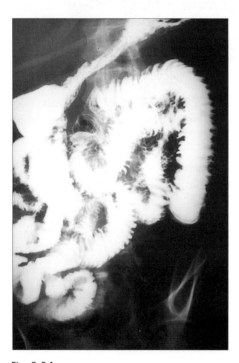

Fig. 3.5.1

Causes of thickened small bowel mucosal folds

- Inflammatory
    Crohn's disease
    Zollinger–Ellison syndrome

- Neoplasia
    lymphoma
    carcinoid
    metastases (esp. melanoma and breast)

- Infection
    tuberculosis
    giardiasis
    strongyloides

- Infiltration
    amyloidosis
    mastocytosis
    eosinophilic enteritis
    Whipple's disease

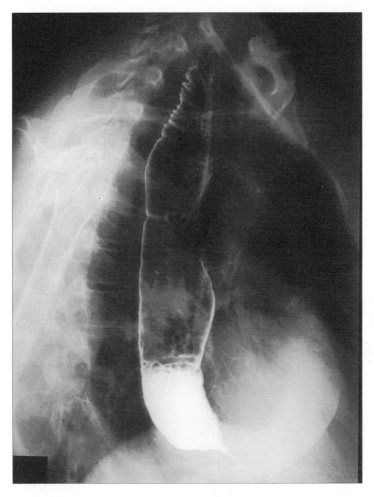

This is a barium swallow of a 52-year-old Caucasian man with a long history of difficulty in swallowing.

A   Describe the abnormality and suggest a diagnosis.
B   What complications may arise?
C   What treatment is available?

ANSWER 3.6

A There is marked dilatation of the oesophagus with a conical narrowing at the cardia ('beak sign'). Residual food debris is evident. The most likely diagnosis is achalasia although it should be noted that Chagas' disease gives an identical picture.

B Complications include the regurgitation of undigested food, which often occurs at night while the patient is recumbent. Recurrent aspiration pneumonia is a common complication (and may be the presenting complaint). Halitosis and nonspecific chest pain may occur. Oesophageal carcinoma develops in 5–10% of patients.

C Medical treatment with nitrates or calcium-channel blockers may be tried.

Endoscopic dilatation of the cardiac sphincter is usually necessary; this relieves symptoms in up to 80% of patients. An open surgical or laparoscopic cardiomyotomy may be required in some patients.

Endoscopy is often readily available but the barium swallow is still a useful investigation in patients with dysphagia. It may demonstrate an oesophageal stricture, which may appear benign (Fig. 3.6.1) or malignant (Fig. 3.6.2), and oesophageal rings, webs, spasm or ulcerative disorders such as oesophagitis secondary to reflux or infection such as candidiasis. The dysphagic symptoms may even be secondary to extrinsic compression of the oesophagus by mediastinal lymphadenopathy, thyroid masses or aneurysms of the thoracic aorta.

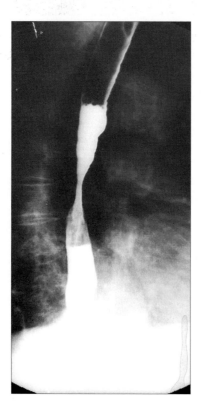

Fig. 3.6.1

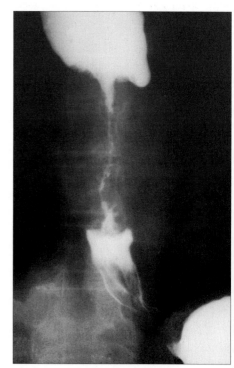

Fig. 3.6.2

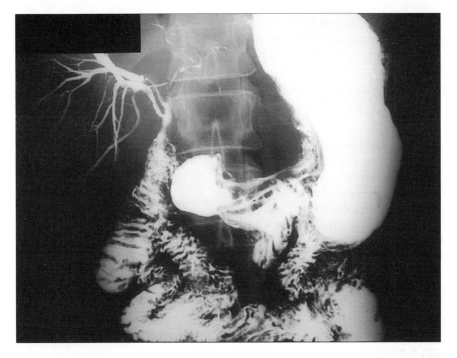

This X-ray is from a barium meal of a 50-year-old man who gives a long history of intermittent upper abdominal discomfort without any previous abdominal surgery.

A Describe the abnormality and suggest an underlying diagnosis.

ANSWER 3.7

A **There is contrast outlining the biliary system indicating the presence of a duodenobiliary fistula. The most common cause for this appearance is the erosion of a gallstone into the duodenum.**

A chronic inflammatory cholecystitis can result in fistula formation into the duodenum. This complication puts patients at risk of developing an ascending cholangitis. If the gallstones are small they may pass through the gut without any untoward events. However, a large gallstone may cause intestinal obstruction. A plain abdominal X-ray may reveal aerobilia (Fig. 3.7.1). Gallstones may also pass into and obstruct the common bile duct (Fig. 3.7.2 – T-tube cholangiogram and Fig. 3.7.3 – helical CT cholangiogram).

Causes of biliary enteric fistulae
● Cholelithiasis (90%)
● Acute/chronic cholecystitis

● Neoplasia
   biliary tract
   invasive bowel tumours

● Inflammatory bowel disease
● Peptic ulcer disease
● Trauma and post-surgery

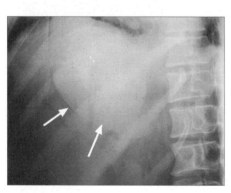

Fig. 3.7.1

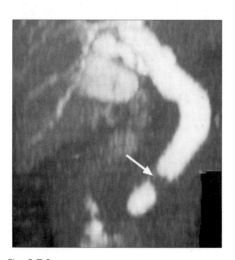

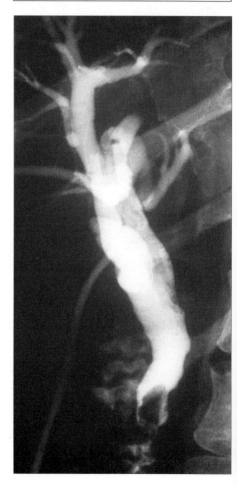

Fig. 3.7.3

Fig. 3.7.2

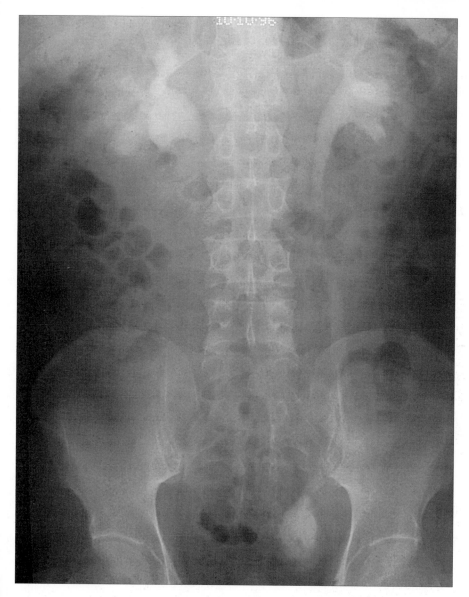

This X-ray is of an intravenous urogram of a 37-year-old man who gives a history of three episodes of right-sided abdominal discomfort associated with fever over the preceding 6 months that have been treated with antibiotics by his general practitioner.

A Describe the abnormalities and suggest an underlying diagnosis.
B What surgical procedure has the patient undergone in the past?
C What further investigation is indicated?

A There is a mild right-sided hydronephrosis whereas the left kidney is normal. The history suggests that the patient has suffered from episodic right-sided pyelonephritis. There is no evidence of a normal bladder. The contrast collects in an indistinct structure. In addition there is a midline fusion defect in the sacrum. This patient has congenital spina bifida.

B This patient has a neurogenic bladder and an ileal conduit has previously been fashioned.

C The right hydronephrosis may be secondary to stenosis of the anastomosis between the right ureter and the conduit, and the investigation of choice is a 'loopogram'. Contrast is instilled through the conduit and should reflux up both ureters and drain freely thereafter. The right kidney does not drain freely in this patient (Fig. 3.8.1).

It is important to scrutinize all of a radiograph for clues as to the underlying diag-

nosis. It should be noted that a stenosis of the ileal conduit would result in bilateral hydronephrosis. The neurogenic bladder has been surgically isolated and is therefore not visualized during these procedures.

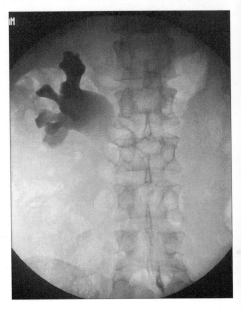

Fig. 3.8.1

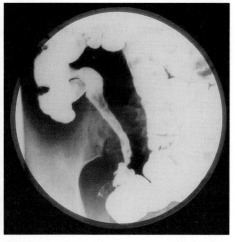

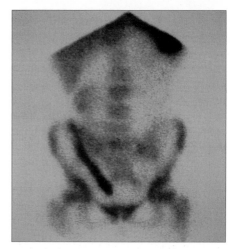

A   B

Film A is of a small bowel enema performed on a 36-year-old man who gives a 9-month history of intermittent abdominal pain, loss of weight and occasional diarrhoea. Film B is of an indium-labelled WBC radioisotope scan of the same patient.

A   Describe the abnormalities and suggest an underlying diagnosis.

B   What treatment is available?

[A] Film A demonstrates the 'string sign'. The thin almost linear collection of barium in the terminal ileum is a result of spasm, ulceration and possibly scarring and is almost pathognomonic of Crohn's disease. The isotope scan reveals increased uptake over the right iliac fossa, reflecting the marked inflammation of the affected portion of bowel.

[B] Treatment includes medical therapy such as sulphasalazine, mesalazine, corticosteroids and immunosuppressive agents such as azathioprine or cyclosporin A. Nutritional support is valuable in some patients, for example low residue diet if intestinal narrowing is present, and vitamin supplementation. Antibiotics such as metronidazole are useful for perianal disease. Abscesses, fistulae and inflammatory or fibrotic strictures may require surgical treatment.

Crohn's disease may affect any part of the gastrointestinal tract. It may therefore be evident in many types of radiological investigations, including barium swallows (ulceration, nodularity and fistulae), barium meals (thickened folds) or small or large bowel enemata (separation of small bowel loops, areas of narrowing or stricture formation [Fig. 3.9.1] or fistulae). Crohn's colitis, which occurs in 15–20% of patients, typically affects the proximal colon unlike ulcerative colitis, which is usually left-sided and distal in location (Fig. 3.9.2). Bowel involvement in Crohn's disease may vary from occasional aphthous ulcers to deep irregular ulceration with fistulae and sinus tracts.

Differential of small bowel strictures

- Crohn's disease
- Adhesions
- Ischaemia (including DXR-related)
- Tumours (lymphoma, carcinoid, primary carcinoma and metastases)
- Tuberculosis

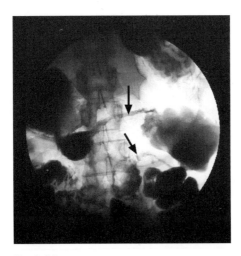

Fig. 3.9.1

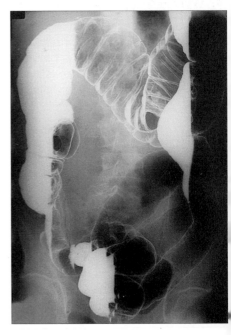

Fig. 3.9.2

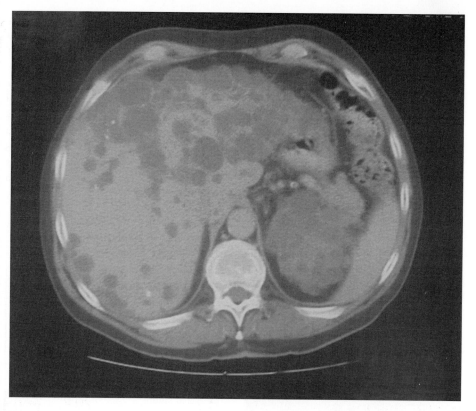

This abdominal CT scan is of a 38-year-old man who is hypertensive and has a strong family history of intracerebral haemorrhage.

A Describe the abnormalities and suggest an underlying diagnosis.
B What treatment is available?
C What further investigation is indicated?

ANSWER 3.10

A There are multiple low-attenuation lesions throughout the liver and the left kidney. The diagnosis is polycystic kidney disease with marked liver involvement.

B These patients are often hypertensive and may well develop renal failure. There is no specific therapy but the meticulous control of hypertension is crucial.

C Cerebral vascular imaging is indicated to exclude an associated intracerebral berry aneurysm. MR-angiography (MRA) is less invasive than bilateral 4-vessel intracerebral angiography and will detect the majority of aneurysms larger than 5 mm in diameter that may well require elective clipping.

Approximately one-third of patients with autosomal dominant polycystic kidney disease (APKD) have hepatic cysts that may vary from minimal involvement to almost complete replacement of the liver parenchyma. Interestingly, however, they do not usually interfere with hepatic function. The diagnosis of APKD is normally made by ultrasound (Fig. 3.10.1) rather than intravenous urography (Fig. 3.10.2). Aspiration of a cyst under ultrasound control may be useful in patients who develop infection or bleeding into a renal or hepatic cyst.

> **APKD associations**
>
> - Cysts – liver, pancreas and occasionally lung, seminal vesicles and thyroid
> - Aneurysms of cerebral vessels (saccular)
> - Mitral valve prolapse
> - Hypertension
> - Renal failure
> - Proteinuria and haematuria

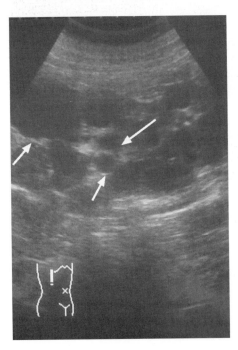

Fig. 3.10.1

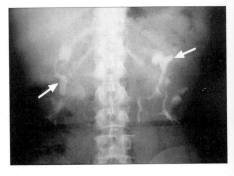

Fig. 3.10.2

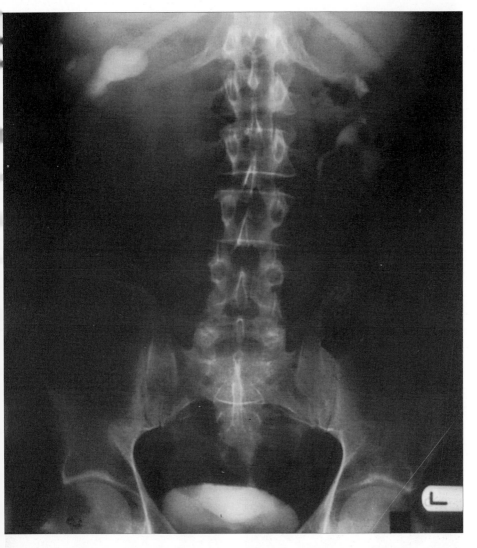

This film is of an intravenous urogram of a 56-year-old man who gives a history of intermittent painless macroscopic haematuria and is found to be mildly hypercalcaemic.

A Describe the abnormality and suggest a diagnosis.
B What further investigations are indicated?
C Suggest two causes for the hypercalcaemia.

ANSWER 3.11

A The left kidney is normal. There is a very large soft-tissue mass, with gross compression and upward displacement of the right pelvicalyceal system. This appearance is very suggestive of a renal cell carcinoma.

B Further investigations include an abdominal CT scan to detect evidence of involvement of the renal vein and para-aortic lymph nodes (Fig. 3.11.1 – different patient) together with an isotope bone scan in view of the hypercalcaemia.

C The hypercalcaemia may be sec-ondary to bony metastases or ectopic production of PTH-like substance by the primary tumour.

Renal cell carcinoma is the most common type of malignant renal neoplasm. Arterio-graphy can demonstrate a hypervascular tumour circulation (Fig. 3.11.2). Tumours may be large and may exhibit calcification (6%) (Fig. 3.11.3). Renal cell carcinomas may produce ectopic hormones, including PTH-like substance, erythropoietin or renin leading to hypercalcaemia, polycythaemia or hypertension, respectively.

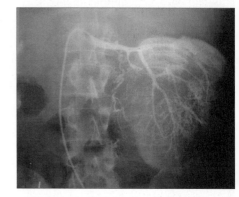

Fig. 3.11.2

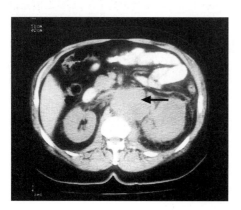

Fig. 3.11.1

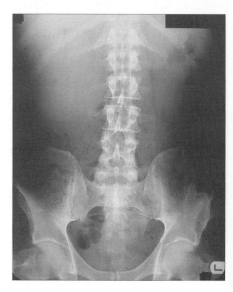

Fig. 3.11.3

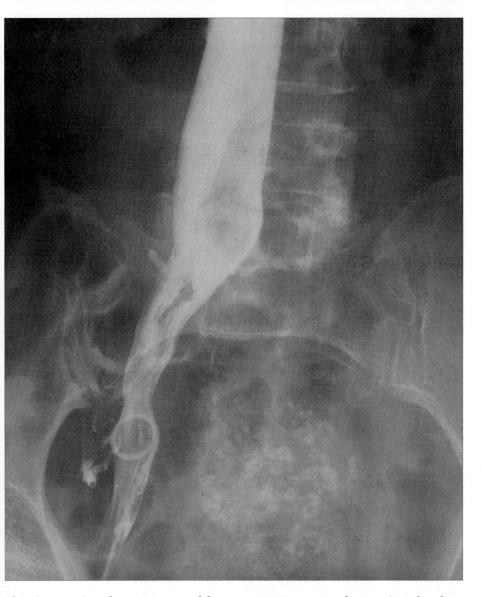

This image is of a 52-year-old woman. One month previously she suffered an acute intracerebral haemorrhage.

A Describe the abnormality.

B Suggest a suitable treatment.

ANSWER 3.12

A This cavogram demonstrates a large clot extending from the left common iliac vein upwards into the inferior vena cava. There is also a pelvic mass with punctate calcification typical of a large calcified fibroid.

B In view of the recent history of intracerebral haemorrhage, anticoagulation would be extremely hazardous. However, the potential of a life-threatening pulmonary embolus requires some form of treatment. The insertion of a caval filter is clinically acceptable.

Indications for the insertion of caval filters (Fig. 3.12.1) include documented extensive free floating thrombus in the iliofemoral veins that is very likely to embolize and significant deep venous thrombosis or documented pulmonary embolic disease in patients in whom anticoagulation is contraindicated, for example patients who have undergone recent surgery, or who have active gastrointestinal bleeding or intracranial haemorrhage. Filters may be left in situ long term or they may be used as a temporary measure and can be percutaneously removed a few weeks later. The main complications of caval filters are misplacement or migration to the right side of the heart, or caval thrombosis.

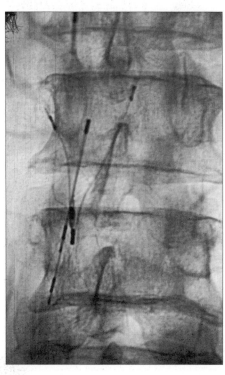

Fig. 3.12.1

Indications for the insertion of caval filters

- Pulmonary embolism (PE) with contraindication to anticoagulation

- Recurrent PE despite adequate anticoagulation

- Deep venous thrombosis with contraindication to anticoagulation

- Deep venous thrombosis in patients with pre-existing pulmonary hypertension

- Post-pulmonary embolectomy

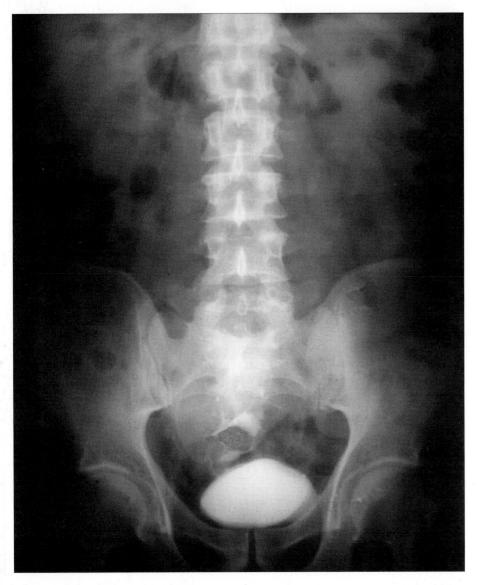

This film is of the intravenous urogram of a 33-year-old man who gave a history of severe intermittent left loin pain.

A Describe the abnormality and suggest a diagnosis.
B What further investigations are indicated?

A There is no contrast evident at either renal area. However, contrast may be seen within the pelvicalyceal system of a single pelvic kidney overlying the sacrum. The other kidney may be congenitally absent or nonfunctional (because of an accompanying obstruction). However, it is more typical for obstructed kidneys to exhibit a delayed and progressively intense nephrogram with dilatation of the pelvicalyceal system and ureter proximal to the obstruction.

B An ultrasound examination is indicated to determine whether a second kidney is present. A urological opinion is required if complete obstruction is demonstrated. Biochemical screening for conditions that predispose to the formation of renal calculi such as hyperparathyroidism, hypercalciuria and hyperuricosuria is indicated. This is particularly important if the patient has a single pelvic kidney as an obstructing renal calculus could cause acute renal failure in this context.

Kidneys may be congenitally absent, ectopic or abnormal. Ectopic kidneys may even lie within the thorax. The horseshoe kidney is the commonest type of fusion abnormality (Fig. 3.13.1). The kidneys are joined at the lower poles by an isthmus of fibrous tissue or normal renal parenchyma. This causes malrotation, which can lead to an appearance similar to pelvicalyceal obstruction although true obstruction may also occur because of the unusual course of the ureter over the isthmus.

A transplant kidney is usually located in either iliac fossa and overlies the ilium. The kidneys may be displaced by marked hepatomegaly or splenomegaly.

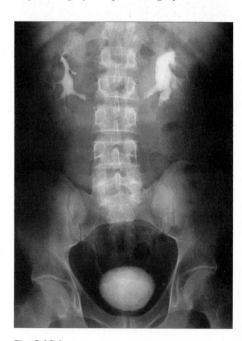

Fig. 3.13.1

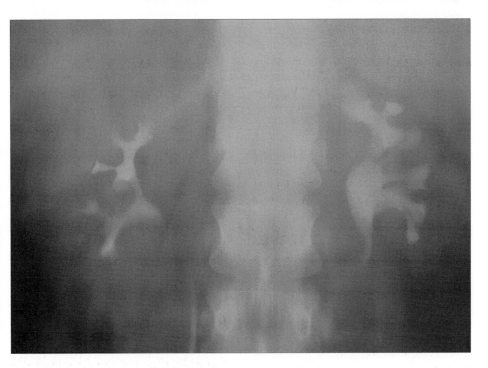

This film (tomogram) is of the intravenous urogram (pregnancy excluded) of a 21-year-old woman who was found to have proteinuria on a routine visit to her general practitioner. Her 24-hour urine protein excretion was 7.4 g.

A Describe the abnormality and give a differential diagnosis.
B What further investigations are indicated?

A The right kidney is normal whereas the left kidney shows clubbing of all the calyces and extensive thinning of the renal cortex. This suggests left chronic pyelonephritis. Unilateral chronic pyelonephritis may produce mild proteinuria (increases in pregnancy) but it does not cause the nephrotic syndrome. The heavy proteinuria must be secondary to intrinsic renal disease affecting the structurally normal right kidney such as minimal change disease, focal segmental glomerulosclerosis, membranous nephropathy (idiopathic or secondary to SLE) or possibly IgA nephropathy (Berger's disease).

B A full serological investigation, including an autoantibody screen, complement levels and immunoglobulins should be performed. She requires a right renal biopsy in order to make a histological diagnosis and institute appropriate therapy.

Chronic pyelonephritis or reflux nephropathy is secondary to a combination of vesico-ureteric reflux with intermittent urinary infection. It may be global or multifocal and result in a small shrunken kidney or be localized causing a focal reduction in renal parenchyma that most typically affects the upper poles. Other causes of a unilateral small kidney include congenital renal dysplasia (Fig. 3.14.1, dysplastic right kidney), longstanding renal ischaemia or obstruction as well as rarer causes such as radiation nephritis. Bilateral small smooth kidneys can result from chronic familial or inflammatory glomerulonephritis, hypertensive nephrosclerosis or widespread intrarenal arteriosclerosis, and may be a late sequelae of renal papillary necrosis or medullary cystic disease. Bilateral smoothly enlarged kidneys may be secondary to severe nephrotic syndrome of any cause, amyloidosis, diabetic glomerulosclerosis, acromegaly or acute interstitial nephritis, which may be secondary to an allergic drug reaction or systemic diseases such as sarcoidosis. Renal size is usually normal in diseases causing acute glomerulonephritis such as Wegener's granulomatosis, SLE or Goodpasture's disease.

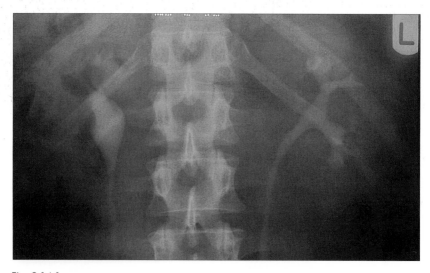

Fig. 3.14.1

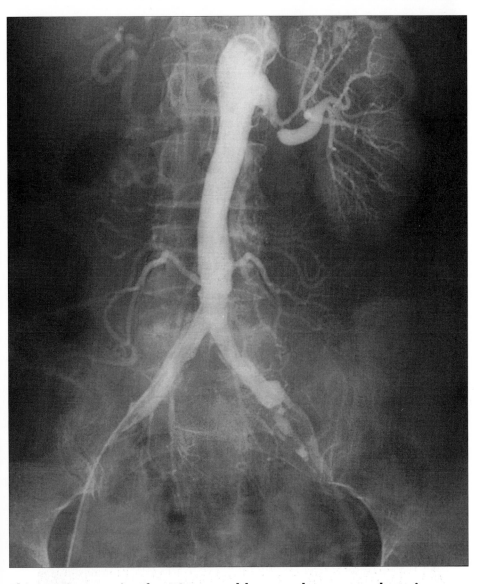

This angiogram is of a 62-year-old man who was undergoing investigations for hypertension.

A Describe the abnormality.
B What potential complications does this investigation have?
C What treatment is available?

ANSWER 3.15

A This angiogram demonstrates a left renal artery stenosis. The right kidney is not visualized either because it is absent or because the right renal artery is completely occluded. This appearance is most likely secondary to atheromatous disease.

B In these patients renal angiography can result in a significant deterioration in renal function secondary to contrast nephropathy (see also Q. 1.1).

C Treatment consists essentially of meticulous control of hypertension although ACE inhibitors must be avoided. A left renal angioplasty may be of benefit and if successful may slow the progression of the otherwise inevitable deterioration to end-stage renal failure.

Renovascular disease is becoming increasingly common in the elderly. It may manifest as hypertension that may be difficult to control with conventional therapy or the patient may develop progressive renal impairment. The stenosis usually occurs in the proximal renal artery and involvement of the ostium is common. Disease may be bilateral in up to one-third of patients. The diagnosis may be suggested from an IVU by the affected kidney being small and irregular with delayed excretion and hyperconcentration of contrast. A renal ultrasound with Doppler is also a useful investigation although spiral CT scanning and MRI are becoming more popular as a less invasive alternative to direct angiography.

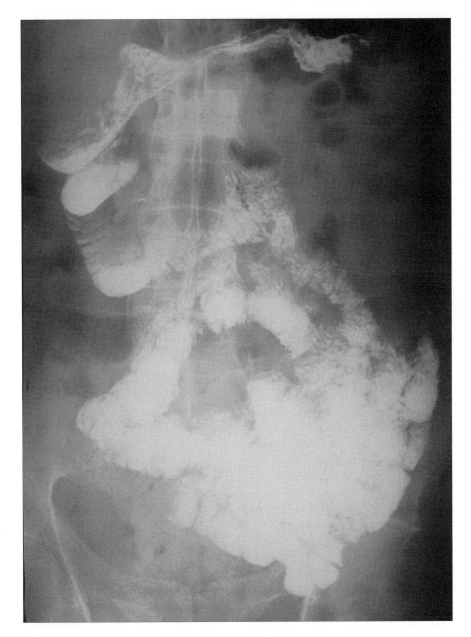

This barium follow through is that of a 41-year-old man.

A Describe the abnormality and suggest a diagnosis and two associated conditions.

B What other organs may be affected?

C What treatment is available?

A This barium follow through is entirely normal. However, there are prominent syndesmophytes in the lumbar spine giving the appearance of a bamboo spine classic of ankylosing spondylitis. Associated conditions include inflammatory bowel disease (though not in this case) and psoriasis.

B Patients with ankylosing spondylitis may develop iritis, upper lobe pulmonary fibrosis, which may cavitate, aortic incompetence and cardiac conduction defects as well as involvement of peripheral joints such as the hip (Fig. 3.16.1) and shoulders, which may necessitate joint replacement. Later complications include a cauda equina syndrome with saddle anaesthesia or secondary amyloidosis.

C Treatment consists of physiotherapy to maintain good posture together with NSAIDs to alleviate stiffness and pain. Indications for second line agents include continued peripheral joint arthritis or a failure to control spinal symptoms in the context of early disease, an elevated acute phase response and an absence of ankylosis on X-ray. Drugs that have been used include sulphasalazine, methotrexate, gold, hydroxychloroquine and steroids. The latter should only be used in short courses and not as long-term therapy. Nocturnal pain may be helped by analgesics, muscle relaxants or amitryptiline.

Ankylosing spondylitis is an inflammatory systemic disease that primarily involves the spine and sacroiliac joints. Plain X-rays may be normal for several years after the onset of symptoms and CT scans and MRI are the most effective early investigations as they may demonstrate early erosive changes in the sacroiliac joints. Isotope scans are more sensitive in these early stages but are non-specific. Radiological features include a bilateral symmetrical and eventually obliterative sacroiliitis and spinal involvement, which initially involves the thoracolumbar junction and then extends. Ossification of spinal ligaments combined with the formation of syndesmophytes leads to a 'bamboo spine' appearance. In long-standing disease osteoporosis and diffuse spinal involvement (Fig. 3.16.2) and calcification of the intervertebral discs may occur. The increased rigidity predisposes to fractures from relatively minor trauma.

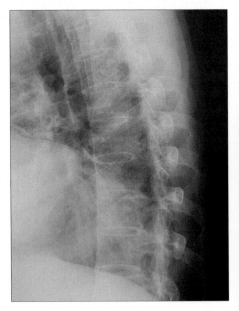

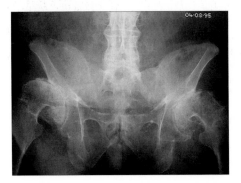

Fig. 3.16.1

Fig. 3.16.2

QUESTION 3.17

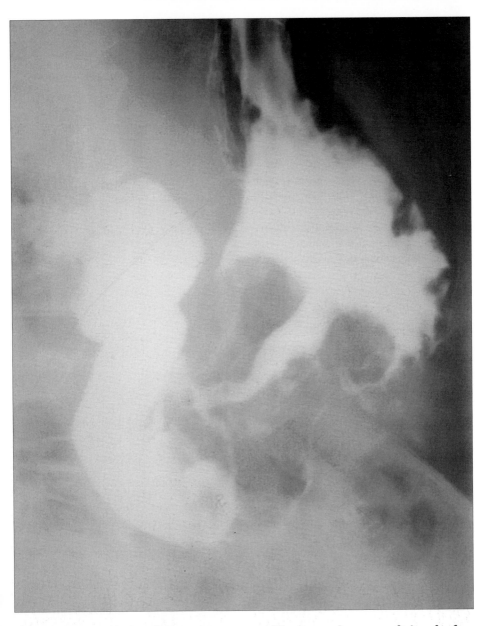

This barium meal is from a 44-year-old man who complained of intermittent abdominal pain and mild anorexia.

A Describe the abnormality and suggest a diagnosis.
B What further investigations are indicated and what treatment is available?

ANSWER 3.17

A There is a large mass within the stomach causing segmental constriction of the gastric body and antrum strongly suggestive of gastric carcinoma.

B This patient requires endoscopy and biopsy of the lesion followed by staging investigations, including routine blood tests and CT scans of the abdomen and chest. Endoscopic ultrasound has also been used to delineate the depth of tumour penetration and lymph node involvement but it is not yet well established. The only potentially curative treatment is surgery but patients often present with advanced disease.

Gastric carcinomas may also give rise to the appearance of linitis plastica ('leather bottle stomach'). The stomach is the commonest site for primary gastrointestinal lymphomas (Fig. 3.17.1), which often lead to marked thickening of the stomach wall. Lymphoma can produce an appearance similar to linitis plastica but stomach wall flexibility and peristalsis are often preserved. Thickening of the gastric folds may be a normal variant (Fig. 3.17.2) but can also be secondary to gastritis, lymphoma, carcinoma, gastric varices or infiltrating conditions such as amyloidosis or Crohn's disease. Barium meals are now less commonly used to diagnose gastric (Fig. 3.17.3) or duodenal ulceration as endoscopy is widely available.

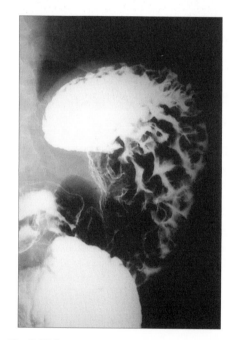

Fig. 3.17.2

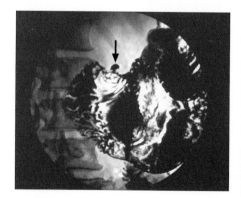

Fig. 3.17.3

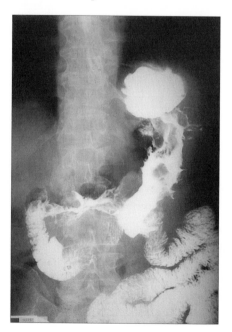

Fig. 3.17.1

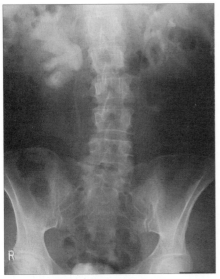

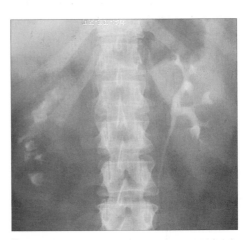

A   **B**

Film A is of the intravenous urogram of a 30-year-old woman who complained of intermittent episodes of right flank pain. Film B was taken 5 minutes after an intravenous injection of frusemide.

A Describe the abnormality and suggest a diagnosis.
B What treatment is available?

A There is marked dilatation of the right renal pelvis but the proximal right ureter is normal in calibre. There is complete emptying after frusemide, which is characteristic of pelviureteric junction (PUJ) obstruction.

B PUJ obstruction is most commonly caused by a failure of peristalsis though it may also be due to extrinsic compression by aberrant blood vessels. Longstanding PUJ obstruction may lead to renal atrophy of the affected kidney and patients may well benefit from an endoluminal or open pyeloplasty.

Imaging investigations play an important role in the investigation and treatment of renal obstruction. Hydronephrosis is readily detectable by ultrasound examination, with dilatation of the renal pelvis and calyceal system (Fig. 3.18.1). An antegrade pyelogram can be performed before the insertion of a draining nephrostomy tube and can delineate the level of obstruction accurately (Fig. 3.18.2). Renal transplant recipients may develop obstruction at any time after surgery (Fig. 3.18.3) and should always undergo an ultrasound examination if the creatinine rises significantly. They can be effectively treated by the radiological insertion of a double J stent. Retrograde pyelography is useful in the investigation of suspected renal pelvis or ureteric malignancy.

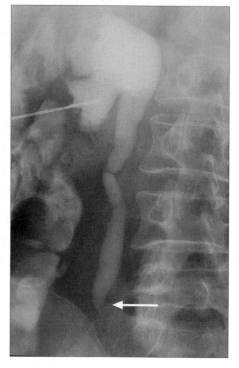

Fig. 3.18.2

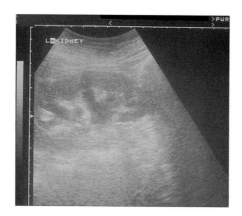

Fig. 3.18.1

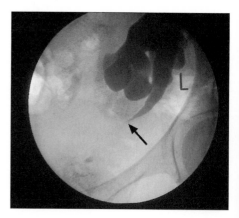

Fig. 3.18.3

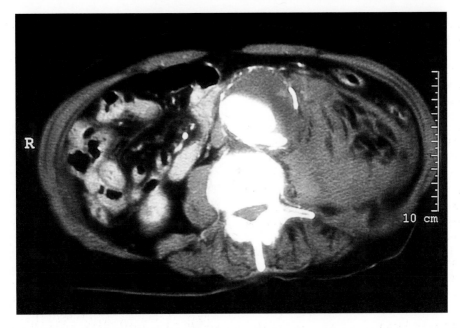

This abdominal CT scan (with contrast) is of a 68-year-old man who has a long history of bilateral calf claudication. He was admitted to hospital with abdominal pain.

A Describe the abnormality and suggest a diagnosis.
B What treatment is available for this condition?

A Contrast can be seen within a markedly dilated abdominal aorta with eccentric peripheral thrombus evident. Adjacent to the aorta is a mass of mixed density that represent an acute retroperitoneal haematoma. This patient has a leaking abdominal aortic aneurysm.

B This patient requires immediate surgical intervention. Patients who have an expanding abdominal aneurysm face elective surgery or, in some instances, may be suitable for stenting of the aneurysm. Figure 3.19.1 and Figure 3.19.2 demonstrate the stent within normal calibre and aneurysmal aorta, respectively.

Percutaneous intravascular stenting procedures are becoming increasingly important and their use can avoid open surgery.

Other examples of conditions amenable to stenting include peripheral vascular disease and renal artery stenosis. Stenting is also useful in obstructive biliary disease (Fig. 3.19.3) and oesophageal carcinoma.

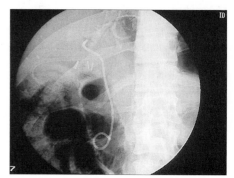

Fig. 3.19.2

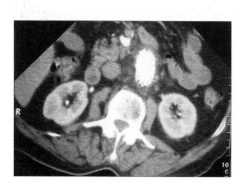

Fig. 3.19.1

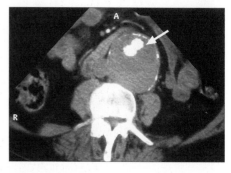

Fig. 3.19.3

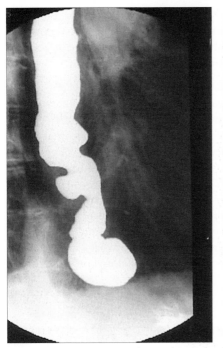 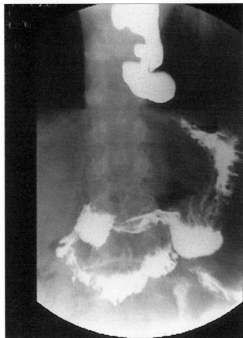

This film is of the barium meal of a 36-year-old man who gives a long history of occasional chest pains and intermittent difficulties in swallowing.

A Describe the abnormality and suggest an underlying diagnosis.
B What treatment is available?

ANSWER 3.20

A The oesophagus demonstrates an abnormal contractile pattern characteristic of the 'cork-screw' oesophagus. This motility disorder typically produces intermittent chest pain and nonprogressive dysphagia for liquids and solids.

B Treatment with calcium-channel blockers or nitrates may be effective, although patients occasionally benefit from oesophageal dilatation.

Barium swallow is still a valuable investigation in patients with difficulties in swallowing. Varied pathologies may be detected, including a pharyngeal pouch (Fig. 3.20.1), an incarcerated hiatus hernia (Fig. 3.20.2), oesophagitis or extrinsic or intrinsic obstructing lesions. It can also give unique information about motility disorders when barium of differing consistencies and soaked solid food (bread) are used to assess for a wide variety of problems (videofluoroscopy).

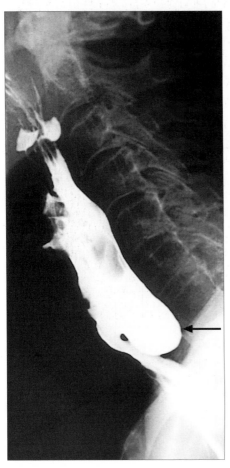

Fig. 3.20.1

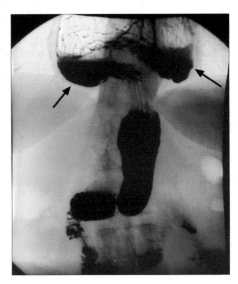

Fig. 3.20.2

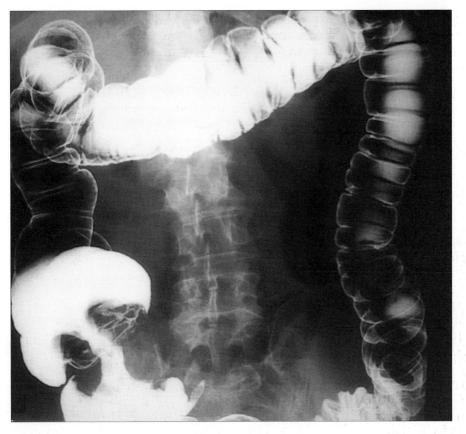

This film is of the barium enema of a 59-year-old man.

A Describe the abnormality and suggest a diagnosis.
B How does the site of the disease affect presentation?
C Give three risk factors for the development of this disease.
D What treatment is available?

ANSWER 3.21

A There is an 'apple core' lesion in the caecum characteristic of an adenocarcinoma (Fig. 3.21.1).

B Tumours of the proximal colon typically manifest with iron deficiency anaemia secondary to occult bleeding whereas tumours of the distal colon manifest with a change of bowel habit or bowel obstruction.

C Risk factors for the development of colorectal cancer include age, a family history of colorectal cancer, a personal history of previous bowel cancer or adenomatous polyps, familial polyposis syndromes and longstanding inflam-matory bowel disease such as ulcerative colitis.

D Treatment consists of surgical re-section with adjuvant chemotherapy and radiotherapy in selected patients. Distal malignant obstructing strictures can (in selected cases) be palliated with a stent procedure.

Barium enema still plays an important role in the investigation of patients with colonic symptoms, demonstrating patho-logies such as diverticular disease and polyps (Fig. 3.21.2). The wide availability of colonoscopy has allowed many patients to be investigated and treated simultane-ously (e.g. the excision/biopsy of polyps).

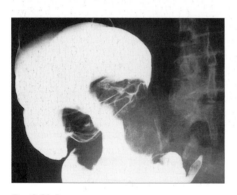

Fig. 3.21.1

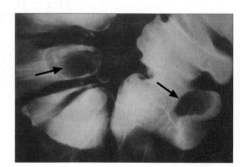

Fig. 3.21.2

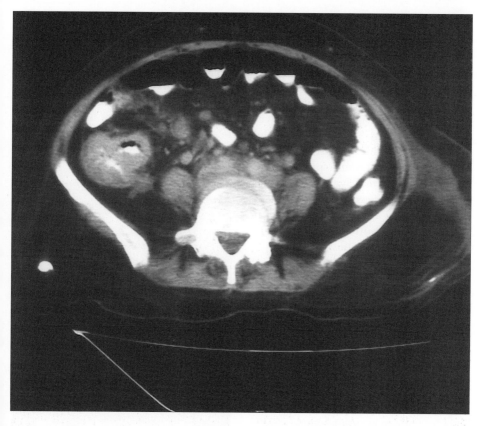

This image is a CT scan through the upper pelvis of a 39-year-old Asian woman. The patient gives a history of weight loss, malaise and occasional fevers and was found to have positive faecal occult blood by her general practitioner.

A Describe the abnormality and give a differential diagnosis.
B What further investigations are indicated?

A The wall of the caecum is markedly thickened and irregular. Adjacent mesenteric lymphadenopathy is also evident (Fig. 3.22.1, lymph node arrowed). This appearance could be a result of inflammatory colitis such as Crohn's disease with reactive lymphadenopathy. Involvement of the distal ileum would be characteristic in this condition. Adenocarcinoma with metastatic spread is also a possibility whereas lymphoma of the large bowel is uncommon. However, this radiological appearance in an Asian patient with intermittent fevers strongly suggests caecal tuberculosis.

B Further investigations include skin testing, chest X-ray (and sputum culture if it is abnormal) and colonoscopy and biopsy (for histology and culture for mycobacteria).

Later in the course of caecal tuberculosis the caecum becomes contracted and narrowed with a patent incompetent ileocaecal valve. Extrapulmonary tuberculosis is not uncommon in various ethnic groups and often is included in the differential diagnosis. The diagnosis is confirmed with isolation and identification of the organism by rhodamine or Ziehl–Neelson staining and culture. The polymerase chain reaction can be used to identify *Mycobacterium tuberculosis* rapidly and differentiate it from other strains. Patients are treated with three to four drugs initially, pending drug sensitivities, with appropriate monitoring for drug toxicity.

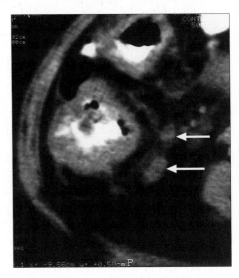

Fig. 3.22.1

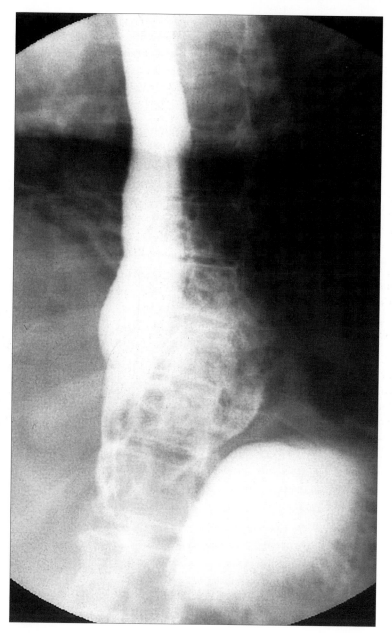

This water-soluble contrast swallow is that of a 29-year-old man who presented to hospital with acute chest pain after a vomiting episode.

A Describe the abnormality and suggest a diagnosis.
B What treatment is indicated?

CONTRAST IMAGES

A There is extensive leakage of contrast into the mediastinum. This patient has a ruptured or perforated oesophagus.

B If possible, conservative treatment (nil orally, antibiotic cover and nutritional support) may suffice. Radiological confirmation of oesophageal healing is mandatory, which may take several weeks.

Specialist thoracic surgical repair is required when mediastinal contamination is extensive. A mediastinal abscess may occasionally be amenable to percutaneous drainage (Figs 3.23.1 and 3.23.2 demonstrate a mediastinal abscess before and after draining respectively).

Causes of oesophageal perforation

- Prolonged or forcible vomiting (Boerhaave's syndrome)
- Closed chest trauma
- Oesophageal instrumentation (including endoscopy)
- Malignancies
- Retained foreign body

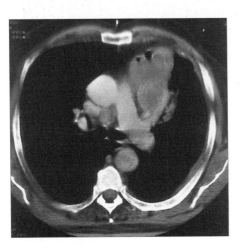

Fig. 3.23.1

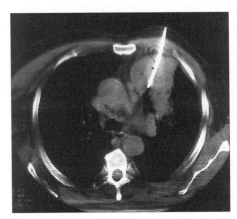

Fig. 3.23.2

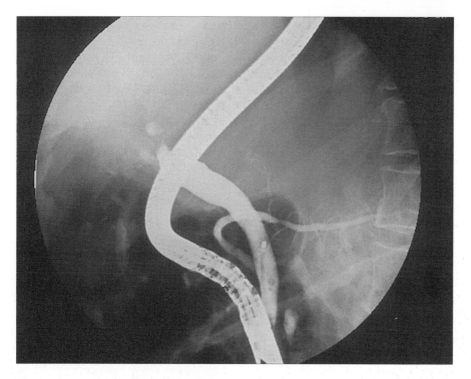

This X-ray is of a 69-year-old woman.

A What is this investigation and what are the complications of the procedure?
B Describe the abnormality and give a differential diagnosis.
C What treatment is available?

A This patient has undergone endoscopic retrograde cholangiopancreatography (ERCP). The main complications of ERCP are acute pancreatitis, biliary sepsis (prophylactic antibiotics required) and haemorrhage (after sphincterotomy).

B The pancreatic duct is normal but there is a tight narrowing of the upper end of the common bile duct. This may be caused by an intrinsic lesion such as a cholangiocarcinoma or extrinsic compression secondary to porta hepatis lymph node enlargement.

C The obstruction may be alleviated by the insertion of a stent to allow biliary drainage.

Ultrasound is the initial imaging investigation of choice in patients with suspected biliary obstruction or gallstones (Fig. 3.24.1) as it is relatively inexpensive and sensitive. ERCP can identify the site and often the nature of biliary obstruction. A papillo-tomy and stone extraction may be performed at the same time as the diagnostic procedure (Fig. 3.24.2). If an ERCP is technically impossible then percutaneous transhepatic cholangiography (PTC) may be performed (Fig. 3.24.3 – PTC needle not visible). Endoscopic ultrasonography is not readily available but is very sensitive at detecting small tumours of the ampulla of Vater or in the head of the pancreas. MRI scanning is increasingly being used to image hepatobiliary pathology.

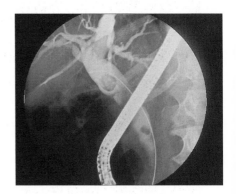

Fig. 3.24.2

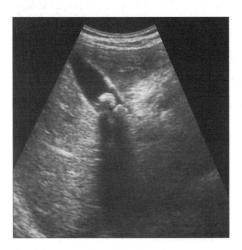

Fig. 3.24.1

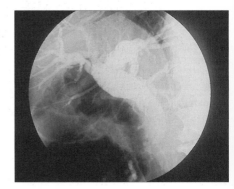

Fig. 3.24.3

QUESTION 3.25

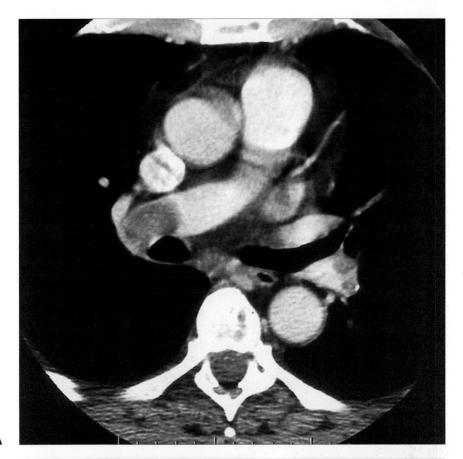

A

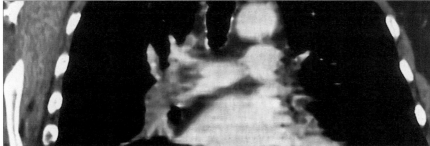

B

Films A and B are of a spiral CT pulmonary angiogram of a 29-year-old woman who is acutely hypoxic. She is currently undergoing investigations for recurrent miscarriages. Routine haematological and biochemical tests have been performed and are unremarkable except for a mild thrombocytopenia.

A Describe the abnormality and suggest an underlying diagnosis.
B What treatment is required?

ANSWER 3.25

A There is a large thrombus in the right pulmonary artery with some smaller left-sided emboli. The history of recurrent miscarriages together with a thrombocytopenia strongly suggests an underlying antiphospholipid antibody syndrome. This may be primary or secondary to systemic lupus erythematosus.

B The mainstay of treatment for pulmonary embolism (PE) is anticoagulation with intravenous heparin followed by oral warfarin. Heparin does not significantly hasten the resolution of established thrombi but does reduce the distal propagation of clot. The activated partial thromboplastin time (APTT) and platelet count should be monitored closely. If the patient is significantly compromised by the pulmonary embolism then thrombolytic therapy should be considered. The insertion of inferior vena cava filters is useful in patients who are at risk of further pulmonary emboli but have a contraindication to anticoagulation. Patients with the antiphospholipid antibody syndrome require long-term anticoagulation.

The chest X-ray may be abnormal in patients with PE. There may be elevation of the hemidiaphragm whereas an area of oligaemia may be evident in the area of the PE (Westermark sign). The pulmonary artery may be prominent and a peripheral pleural-based homogenous wedge-shaped density pointing towards the hilum may be seen if the lung undergoes infarction (Hampton's hump). A normal isotope perfusion scan excludes a significant PE. Ventilation/perfusion (V/Q) scans are labelled as low, intermediate or high probability of PE. A high probability scan (Fig. 3.25.1) has two or more large (or four or more moderate) segmental perfusion defects without corresponding ventilation defects (or significantly smaller ventilation defects) or abnormalities on the chest X-ray. Such a scan merits treatment. V/Q scans of low or intermediate probability are more problematical as up to one-third of patients with such scans will have pulmonary emboli on pulmonary angiography. Therefore such patients are often investigated further to identify the potential site(s) of venous thrombus. These may be noninvasive such as ultrasonography (including Doppler techniques) and impedance plethysmography. Invasive studies (contrast venography) is often performed if noninvasive tests are equivocal.

Practice between centres may vary considerably and reflects local expertise, availability, and access to individual techniques.

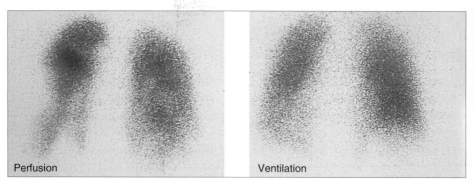

Perfusion

Ventilation

Fig. 3.25.1

HEAD AND NECK RADIOLOGY

Introduction: head and neck radiology

The head and neck is mainly investigated utilising cross-sectional imaging. Plain films are still used and ultrasound is extremely useful for assessing structures such as the salivary, thyroid and parathyroid glands and lymph nodes, particularly with a view to image-guided biopsy.

In assessing plain skull radiographs, consider the following:

- Bones: calvarial thickness; local areas of diminished bone density or erosions, size of sella (depth 5 to 11 mm; length 7 to 12 mm).
- Soft tissues.
- Sinuses: opaque; fluid levels.
- Intraorbital or intracranial gas shadow.
- Calcification: often physiological in choroid plexus, pineal gland, falx, tentorium and clinoid ligaments. Abnormal causes include congenital (often due to infection), vascular and neoplastic.
- Linear translucencies may be normal: vascular channels.
- Evidence of bone softening: basilar invagination indicated by elevated odontoid peg (>6mm above McGregor's line between the lowermost point of the external occiput to back of hard palate) with a Bull's angle subtended between line through atlas and line of hard palate > 13 degrees).

As with other body regions cross-sectional imaging investigations are rarely interpreted by clinicians without the aid of a radiologist. For the purposes of the diploma examination candidates should be aware of certain appearances, particularly on CT, in relation to causes of acute neurological deterioration. These include subarachnoid, subdural, extradural and intracerebral haemorrhage and cerebral infarction. Acute haemorrhage is of high attenuation (appears dense) on unenhanced scans. One should be familiar with potential causes of mass lesions: primary or secondary neoplasms and infective foci.

In assessing cranial CT, consider the following:

- Ventricular size and symmetry. Appearance in relation to sulci, which become more apparent with age.
- Presence of intracranial abnormality: extra-axial (outwith the brain substance) or intra-axial (arising from within the brain parenchyma).
- Space-creating (atrophy focal or generalised) or space-taking (mass) lesion.
- Single or multiple lesion(s).
- Physical characteristics of abnormality: shape and margin/composition/density; response to intravenous contrast.
- Skull: shape and thickness.
- Appearance of sinuses and mastoid air cells – presence of opacification.

MRI is utilised widely in neuroradiology. Its multiplanar capability enables further characterisation of abnormalities and is of particular use in imaging the posterior fossa where CT is limited due to artefact arising from bone in the skull base. Detailed understanding of MRI is not required. Essentially, based on the response of their hydrogen nuclei, different tissues exhibit different physical properties (T1 and T2) when placed in a superconducting magnet after exposure to a series of electromagnetic pulses at predetermined time intervals. These differential properties are exploited by setting parameters (TE – time to echo; TR – time to repeat) that elicit images based on the T1 or T2 properties of the tissue.

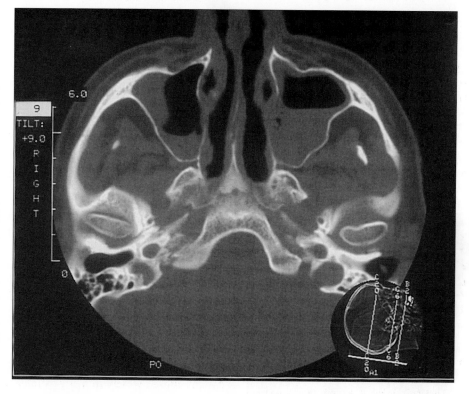

This CT scan is of a 47-year-old man who has recently returned from Spain where he was unwell with an 'atypical pneumonia'. He now presents to hospital with haemoptysis and has microscopic haematuria and proteinuria.

A Describe the abnormality.
B Suggest a diagnosis.
C What other investigations should be performed?

A There is a bilateral maxillary sinusitis with marked mucosal thickening and an air-fluid level on the left, but no bony erosion.

B The combination of sinusitis, haemoptysis and dipstick haematuria and proteinuria suggests a diagnosis of Wegener's granulomatosis. This is a multisystem granulomatous small vessel vasculitis that typically affects the upper and lower respiratory tracts together with the kidneys.

C Required investigations include a chest X-ray (patients may have cavitating pulmonary granulomata or alveolar haemorrhage), measurement of oxygen saturation and arterial blood gases if hypoxic, urea and electrolytes, urine microscopy for casts and serum should be sent for an urgent antineutrophil cytoplasmic antibody assay (ANCA). A histological diagnosis is required and a biopsy of involved tissues (nose, lung or kidney) should be performed. The characteristic histological finding is the presence of noncaseating granulomata.

Involvement of the sinuses in Wegener's granulomatosis may vary from mild soft-tissue swelling or polypoidal lesions to extensive bony destruction. Other destructive lesions that may involve the sinuses include sarcoidosis, midline granuloma and squamous cell carcinomas (which mainly arise in the maxillary sinuses).

The combination of sinus disease (Fig. 4.1.1) with dextrocardia and bronchiectasis is found in Kartagener's syndrome (Fig. 4.1.2, previous left upper thoractomy).

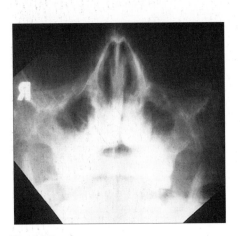

Fig. 4.1.1

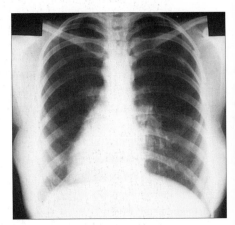

Fig. 4.1.2

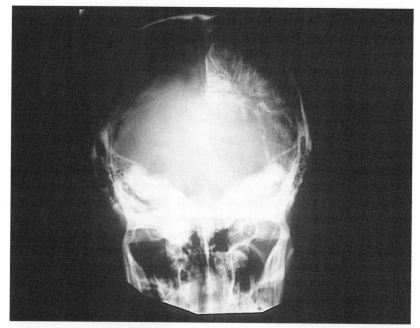

A

B

Films A and B are skull X-rays of a 30-year-old man.

A Describe the abnormality.
B Suggest a diagnosis and describe the associated clinical features.

A There is spectacular occipital 'tram-line' calcification.

B Sturge–Weber syndrome (encephalo-facial angiomatosis). Associated features include a port-wine naevus on the ipsilateral side of the face (often in the distribution of the trigeminal nerve) and epilepsy. Affected individuals may also have glaucoma, exophthalmos, optic atrophy or a squint.

In the Sturge–Weber syndrome the calcification is within the brain cortex and underlies the pial angiomatosis. It most commonly involves the parieto-occipital region. The calcification seems to undulate and follow the contours of the brain surface.

Intracranial calcification affecting the pineal gland (Fig. 4.2.1), dura, basal ganglia and choroid plexus may be normal. Solitary intracranial calcification may occur in vascular malformations and aneurysms, neoplasms such as meningiomas, gliomas or craniopharyngiomas, and more rarely in chronic subdural haematomas and areas of scarring such as old cerebral infarcts. Multiple intracranial calcifications may result from infectious diseases such as congenital cytomegalovirus (CMV) or toxoplasma infection, cysticercosis, tuberculosis, meningitis, paragonimiasis or hydatid disease. Patients with tuberous sclerosis (Bourneville's disease) develop calcified nodules along the wall of the ventricles and the disease is complicated by a giant cell astrocytoma in about 10% of patients (Fig. 4.2.2, calcified nodules and asterocytoma indicated by arrowheads and arrow, respectively). The tubers or tumour may also cause an obstructive hydrocephalus.

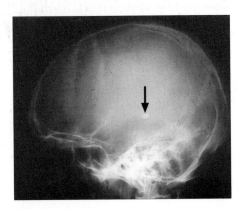

Fig. 4.2.1

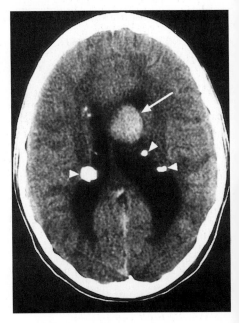

Fig. 4.2.2

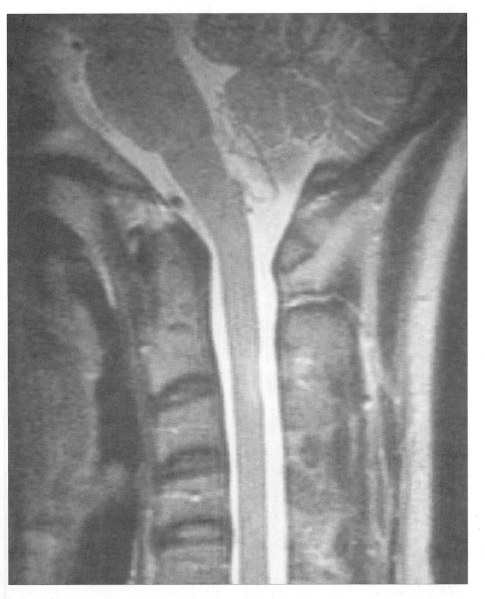

This MRI scan is of a 34-year-old man with a 4-month history of weakness of his left leg.

A Describe the abnormality and suggest the most likely diagnosis.
B What treatment is available?

A There is an area of increased signal at the C2–3 level that is characteristic of an area of damaged myelin. This patient probably has multiple sclerosis.

B Spasticity may be helped by baclofen and benzodiazepines whereas bladder dysfunction may require anticholinergic drug therapy and/or intermittent self-catheterization (exclude UTI and consider urodynamic testing). Neuralgic symptoms may respond to carbamazepine or amitryptiline. High-dose intravenous methylprednisolone followed by a short course of oral prednisone has been demonstrated to hasten the recovery from acute exacerbations of multiple sclerosis. Steroids should only be given to patients who experience a demonstrable functional impairment as a result of the exacerbation and should not be given simply for fluctuations in symptomatology. Recently treatment with recombinant human beta-interferon has been shown to reduce significantly the frequency of exacerbations, the development of demyelination plaques (as demonstrated by MRI scan) and the rate of disease progression.

Plaques of demyelination produce areas of increased signal on T2-weighted MRI scans. In the spinal cord plaques are characteristically located peripherally and are not extensive. The spinal cord may be swollen acutely whereas in longstanding lesions spinal cord atrophy may develop. A similar appearance can be found in patients with a transverse myelitis or the AIDS-related myelopathy. However, these lesions tend to be more diffuse and larger. Approximately two-thirds of patients who present with a myelopathy will have multiple lesions evident on an MRI scan of the brain. These typically occur in the periventricular regions (Fig. 4.3.1, example arrowed). Acute lesions may enhance as shown on T1-w sequences after gadolinium contrast administration (Fig. 4.3.2, example arrowed). High-signal lesions in the periventricular white matter also occur in cerebral ischaemia, migraine, cerebral vasculitides and after radiation therapy.

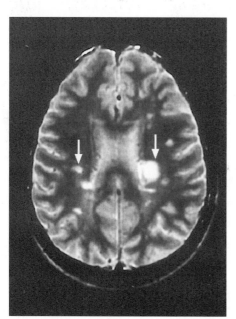

Fig. 4.3.1

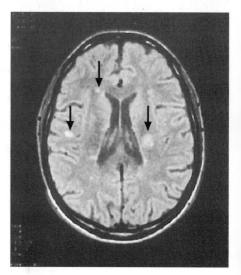

Fig. 4.3.2

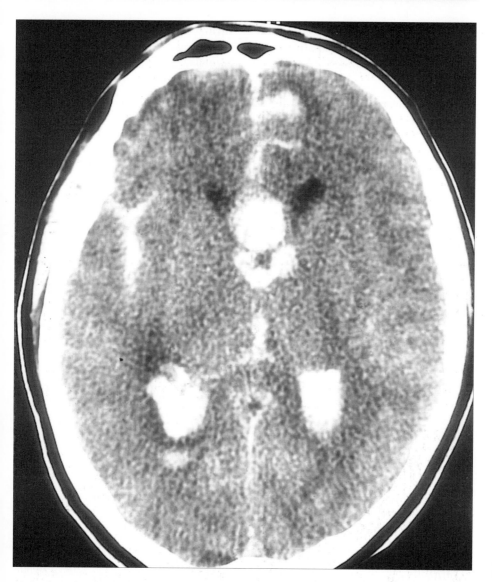

This unenhanced CT scan is of a 44-year-old woman who was admitted unconscious to hospital.

A Describe the abnormality and suggest a diagnosis.
B She rapidly developed respiratory distress after admission. Suggest two causes.

ANSWER 4.4

A There is extensive blood within the ventricular system indicative of a subarachnoid haemorrhage.

B Concomitant respiratory distress is usually secondary to either noncardiogenic pulmonary oedema or aspiration.

Causes of subarachnoid haemorrhage include hypertension and structural lesions such as aneurysms (Fig. 4.4.1) or arteriovenous malformations (Fig. 4.4.2). MRI is becoming increasingly useful in the detection of these lesions. For example, patients with autosomal dominant polycystic kidney disease who have a strong family history of cerebral haemorrhage may be screened for the presence of associated berry aneurysms by MR-angiography.

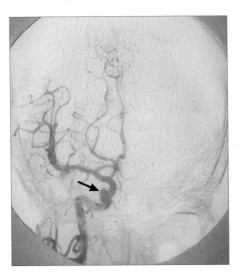

Fig. 4.4.1

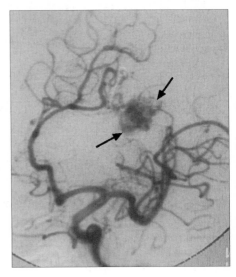

Fig. 4.4.2

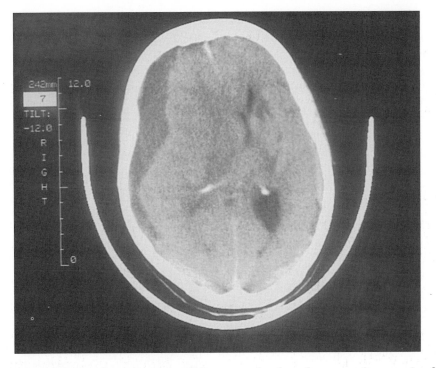

This CT scan is of a 64-year-old man who has become increasingly vague and disorientated since a minor road traffic accident 3 weeks earlier.

A Describe the abnormality and suggest a diagnosis.
B Outline treatment.

ANSWER 4.5

A There is a roughly crescentic low attenuation region in the right fronto-parietal area, with significant compression of the right ventricular system and midline shift from right to left. This is a subdural haematoma with significant mass effect.

B These patients should be managed jointly with the neurosurgeons. Surgical evacuation of the haematoma combined with general supportive care is often indicated but this depends upon the general condition of the patient.

CT scanning is indicated in patients who have suffered an acute neurological event. A subdural haematoma may be acute or chronic and usually results from bleeding from the veins between the dura and the leptomeninges. An acute subdural haematoma is a peripheral high attenuation crescentic lesion and blood may be present in the interhemispheric fissure (Fig. 4.5.1). Over a period of several weeks the attenuation of the collection falls such that it becomes isodense and then hypodense. Subdural haematomata may be bilateral (Fig. 4.5.2). Acute intracerebral haemorrhage (Fig. 4.5.3) produces a high-density intracerebral mass on plain scans. Accurate diagnosis in such patients is important so that potentially beneficial neurosurgical evacuation of haematomas can be undertaken with minimal delay.

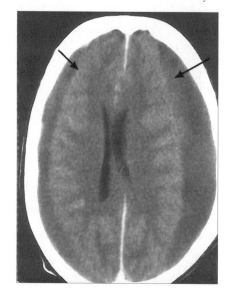

Fig. 4.5.2

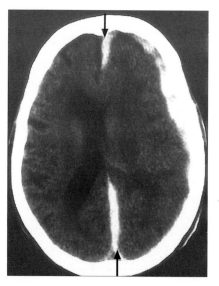

Fig. 4.5.1

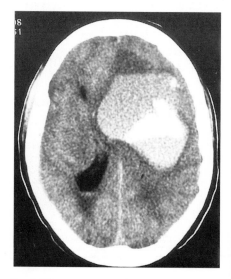

Fig. 4.5.3

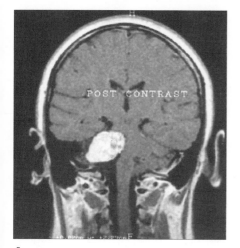

A

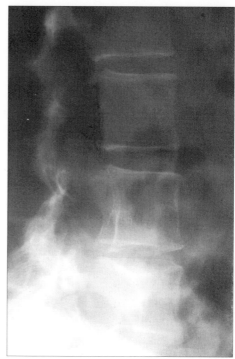

B

Film A is an MRI scan of a 40-year-old man who complains of an unsteady gait and unilateral sensorineural deafness. Film B is an X-ray (of a different patient) arranged by his general practitioner because of mild low-back pain.

A Describe the abnormalities and suggest a unifying diagnosis for these different patients.

B What clinical signs may be present?

C Outline treatment.

ANSWER 4.6

A In film A there is a large enhancing lesion in the cerebellopontine region, with significant displacement of the adjacent brainstem.

In film B there is scalloping of the posterior vertebral bodies. These patients demonstrate some of the differing manifestations of the spectrum of neurofibromatosis.

B Patients may have palpable cutaneous neurofibromas (which may be plexiform),

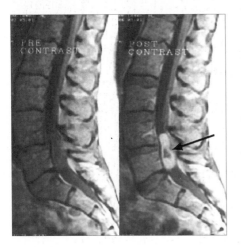

Fig. 4.6.1

axillary freckles and cafè au lait spots. Patients are more likely to develop a phaeochromocytoma and a scoliosis.

C There is no effective treatment for the underlying condition but tumours may well need to be surgically excised.

Neurofibromatosis is a neurocutaneous disorder that may be autosomal dominant or arise sporadically. Patients have an increased risk of tumours, including acoustic neuromas (which may be bilateral) and neurofibromas, which may involve other cranial or spinal nerves (Fig. 4.6.1). Tumours may be evident on plain X-rays (Fig. 4.6.2).

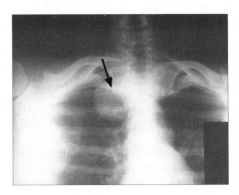

Fig. 4.6.2

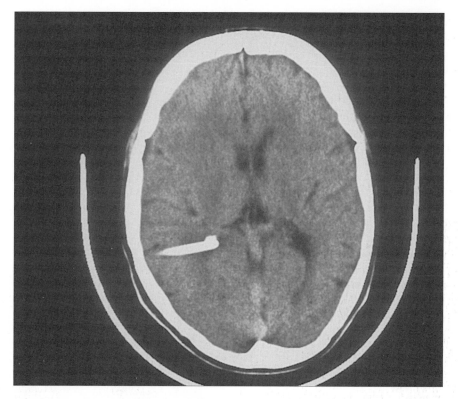

This CT scan is of a 26-year-old man who presented to hospital feeling generally unwell with a fever. He had mild pedal oedema and mild renal impairment with haematuria and proteinuria on dipstix. His blood pressure was 190/100.

A Describe the abnormality and suggest an underlying diagnosis.
B Outline investigations and treatment.

A There is a shunt present but no evidence of increased intracranial pressure. The patient is hypertensive and fluid overloaded, with renal impairment indicating nephritis. The history and presence of an intracranial shunt suggests a shunt infection complicated by a secondary glomerulonephritis.

B After multiple cultures the patient should be treated with intravenous broad spectrum antibiotics. A neurosurgical opinion should be sought regarding the necessity and timing of shunt replacement. Further investigations include serum immunoglobulins, complement and cryoglobulin levels, urine microscopy for casts and a renal ultrasound and echocardiogram. Treatment includes salt restriction, careful fluid balance and possibly diuretics. If there is any doubt that the renal disease is actually unrelated to the infection then antineutrophil cell antibody (ANCA) and antiglomerular basement membrane antibody levels should be determined and a renal biopsy performed in order to obtain a histological diagnosis.

CT scanning is very useful in the investigation of suspected intracerebral infection. A cerebral abscess typically has a hypodense central zone surrounded by a thin ring. There is a uniform ring of enhancement with contrast administration (Fig. 4.7.1). Hydatid cysts are sharply demarcated and hypodense, while in herpes simplex encephalitis there are poorly defined areas of low attenuation in the temporal and parietal lobes. Infection within the ventricular system can result in the typical appearance of 'ventriculitis' (Fig. 4.7.2). Calcification may be evident within healed tuberculomas (Fig. 4.7.3).

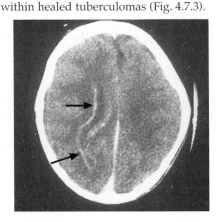

Fig. 4.7.2

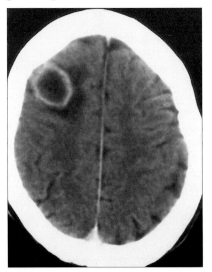

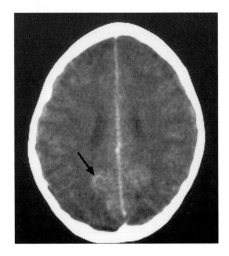

Fig. 4.7.1

Fig. 4.7.3

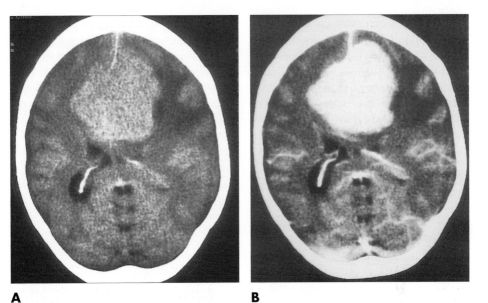

A   **B**

Films A (pre-contrast) and B (post-contrast) are CT scans of a 53-year-old man who gave a history of gradually worsening headaches and presented acutely to hospital after an epileptic fit.

A   Describe the abnormality and suggest a diagnosis.
B   Outline treatment.

A Film A demonstrates a large high-attenuation interhemispheric frontal mass. In film B the mass exhibits intense and homogenous enhancement after administration of contrast. There is minimal cerebral oedema in relation to the large size of the lesion. This appearance is classic of a meningioma.

B The patient should be treated with anticonvulsants and a neurosurgical opinion should be obtained.

CT scanning is indicated in patients who have symptoms or signs of raised intra-cranial pressure. Detectable pathology includes primary brain tumours such as gliomas (Fig. 4.8.1 'butterfly' glioma of anterior corpus callosum) or metastatic secondary deposits (Fig. 4.8.2).

Multiplanar MRI can also give increased anatomical information about adjacent bony and vascular structures to assess surgical operability (Figs 4.8.3 [meningioma] and 4.8.4 [inoperable left temporal cystic astrocytoma]).

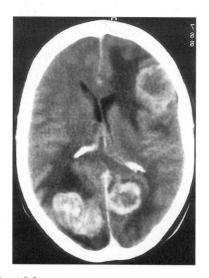

Fig. 4.8.1

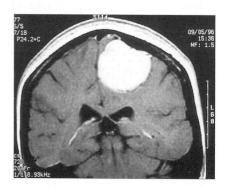

Fig. 4.8.3

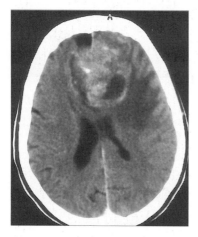

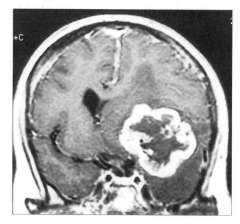

Fig. 4.8.2

Fig. 4.8.4

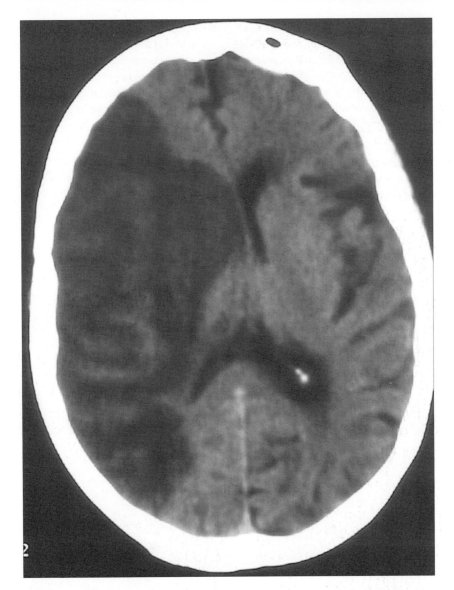

This CT scan is of a 62-year-old woman who collapsed while at work.

A Describe the abnormality and suggest a diagnosis.
B What clinical signs may be present?
C Suggest three possible causes.

A There is a large well defined area of hypodensity that involves the cerebral cortex and the underlying white matter. This is the territory supplied by the right middle cerebral artery and this patient has suffered a complete right middle cerebral artery infarct.

B Middle cerebral artery occlusion produces a contralateral motor and sensory loss and a homonymous hemianopia. If the dominant hemisphere is involved then the patient may be aphasic.

C Potential causes include cerebral atherosclerosis, hypotension, and a cerebral embolic event. Less common causes include thrombotic disorders such as the antiphospholipid antibody syndrome, hyperviscosity states such as polycythaemia and cerebral vasculitides such as temporal arteritis.

The features of an infarct are characteristic. The first radiological sign is obliteration of the normal cerebral sulci with low density of the involved grey and white matter in the infarcted area. More than one artery may be involved as in Figure 4.9.1 where there is simultaneous ischaemic infarction of the right anterior cerebral and right middle cerebral arteries.

The exclusion of acute intracranial haemorrhage enables patients to be considered for anticoagulation treatment. The role of thrombolytic therapies is presently being considered.

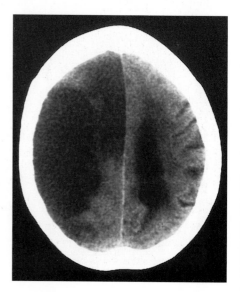

Fig. 4.9.1

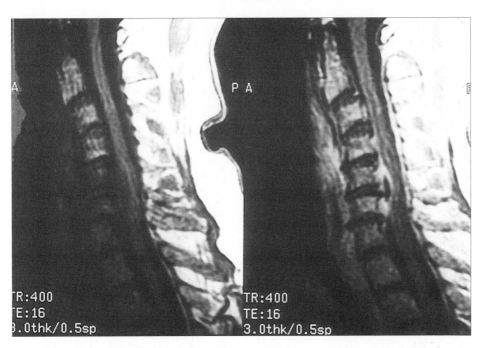

This 55-year-old man had a 4-day history of severe sore throat. He became acutely unwell with severe neck stiffness and pain and upper and lower limb weakness. These sagittal T1-w cervical spine scans are before and after gadolinium contrast administration.

A Describe the imaging findings.
B Suggest a possible diagnosis.
C What additional pathology should be considered?
D What would comprise your immediate management?

ANSWER 4.10

A There is an ellipsoid enhancing lesion in the epidural space anteriorly in the spinal canal at the C5–6 level. The adjacent bone and disc are unremarkable. Considerable compromise of the spinal canal is present, with cord compression.

B These are the appearances of an acute epidural abscess. The acute history and associated symptoms of infection exclude slow-growing tumours as an alternative diagnosis. There is no evidence of an infective discitis or vertebral osteomyelitis.

C This is an unusual acute septic event and as such an underlying immuno-compromising condition should be considered. This illness was the acute and dramatic presentation of insulin-dependent diabetes mellitus. The source of infection was the pharyngitis and method of spread haematogeneous to the spinal venous plexus.

D This patient needs the immediate expert surgical skills of a spinal surgeon for abscess drainage and cord decompression.

Most cases of spinal sepsis have a more chronic history and involve the thoracic and lumbar regions. There is often evidence of disc and bone involvement on plain films (Fig. 4.10.1) and other imaging techniques. MRI scanning is the best investigation to allow the full extent of disc, bony and adjacent soft-tissue involvement to be assessed (Fig. 4.10.2, abnormal bone and soft tissue signal changes D12/L1; plain films were normal).

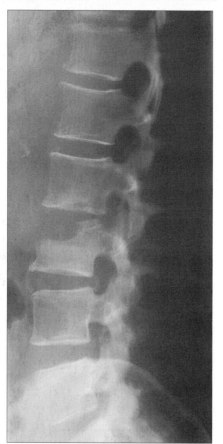

Fig. 4.10.1

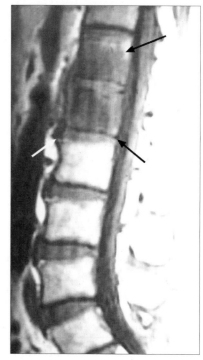

Fig. 4.10.2

THORACIC RADIOLOGY

Introduction: thoracic radiology

The plain chest radiograph (CXR) is the most frequently performed radiographic examination on patients with suspected or known general medical conditions. As in other body regions cross sectional imaging has been shown to further delineate abnormalities demonstrated on plain films and also outline abnormalities not apparent on plain films. CT has a well established role both in conventional scanning in assessing complex structures/masses and in high resolution scanning (thinner sections which demonstrate lung parenchymal architecture). MRI is being increasingly used, particularly in oncology patients. Those suspected of having pulmonary embolic disease in most institutions are investigated by ventilation/perfusion nuclear medicine scan with an increasing role for CT and MRI pulmonary angiography.

Management decisions following interpretation of CXR are often made prior to formal reporting by a radiologist. Familiarity with some technical aspects and the appearances of several disease processes which may be apparent on a CXR is essential.

Technical factors can significantly alter the appearance of the plain chest radiograph. These should be taken into consideration when making an interpretation.

- The projection is defined by the direction the X-ray beam passes through the patient: anteroposterior (AP) or posteroanterior (PA). PA films are taken with the X-ray machine behind the patient and film in front which is the standard projection. AP films which are taken with the X-ray machine in front of the patient and the film at the back result in the heart and other mediastinal structures appearing relatively large. AP films may be taken outside the X-ray department at the patient's bedside.
- Penetration. Posterior ribs should be just visible through the heart shadow.
- Inspiratory effort. At full inspiration the right hemidiaphragm lies between the anterior aspects of the fifth and seventh ribs; the left hemidiaphragm is lower than the right.
- Rotation. Check the positions of the medial ends of the clavicles in relation to the thoracic spinous processes.

A large amount of information is presented on a chest radiograph. Several aspects should be studied. A suggested approach is:

1. Technical factors including projection: AP — medial ends of clavicles tend to be higher than lateral ends and anterior ends of ribs tend to be magnified; PA — lower medial ends of clavicles and smaller anterior ends of ribs

2. Side marker. Is there dextrocardia?

3. Heart. The maximum diameter of the heart should be less than half of the transthoracic diameter.

4. Hilar regions (size, density and relative positions).

5. Lung fields (opacification or lucency).

6. Mediastinal contour.

7. Trachea (position and shape).

8. Bones (see Section 2).

9. Diaphragms. The right hemidiaphragm lies below the level of the anterior end of the 6th rib.

10. Below the diaphragms (free gas, calcified viscera).

11. Soft-tissues (breast shadows, calcification, subcutaneous emphysema).

12. 'Hidden regions' (apices, behind the clavicles, behind the heart, behind the diaphragms and costophrenic angles).

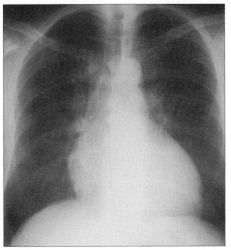

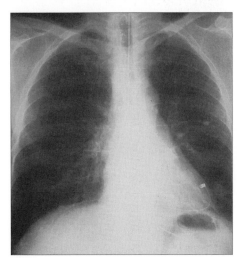

A

B

Film A is a chest X-ray of a 46-year-old man with severe heart disease. Film B is a chest X-ray of the same man after he had undergone treatment in 1990.

A　What treatment has been performed?

B　What complications may arise?

ANSWER 5.1

A Film A demonstrates cardiomegaly whereas in film B the cardiac size is normal and the lung fields are clear. Median sternotomy sutures are evident as is the tip of an epicardial pacing wire. This impressive reduction in cardiac size is not compatible with coronary artery bypass grafting and the patient has undergone a cadaveric cardiac transplant.

B As in all allografts one of the main complications is rejection, which is usually asymptomatic and diagnosed by endomyocardial biopsy. Immuno-suppressed patients are more prone to develop acute and chronic infections and, in the long term, malignancy, particularly lymphomas.

A similar appearance may follow a ventriculectomy but this procedure was not performed in 1990. Drainage of a peri-cardial effusion (Fig. 5.1.1) can also result in the restoration of a normal cardiac silhouette.

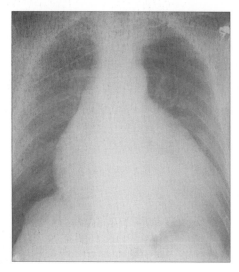

Fig. 5.1.1

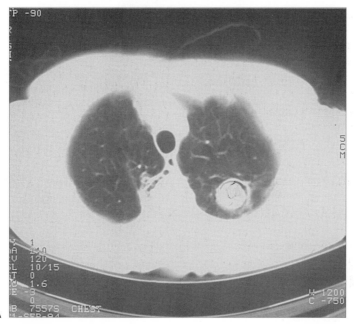

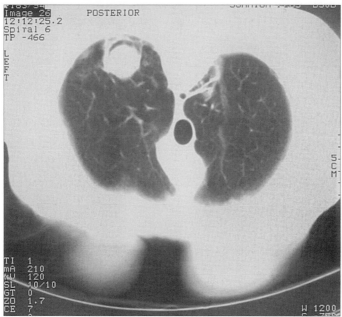

Films A and B are CT scans of a 61-year-old woman.

A Describe the abnormality and suggest a diagnosis.
B What symptoms may be complained of?
C What treatment is available?

ANSWER 5.2

A There is a rounded, smooth mass surrounded by a meniscus of air within a cavity in the upper left lung. In scan A the crescent of air is anterior to the mass whereas in scan B the patient has been turned over and the air is still anterior in location indicating that the mass is mobile. This appearance is typical of a fungus ball or mycetoma, most commonly an aspergilloma, within an old tuberculous cavity.

B Mycetomas may be asymptomatic though haemoptysis commonly occurs. Serum aspergillus precipitins are strongly positive.

C Antifungal treatments are usually ineffective. Intervention may be neces-sary for severe recurrent haemoptysis and may involve surgical resection or bronchial artery embolization.

The majority of fungus balls are caused by *Aspergillus* but they can also result from candidal, nocardial, cryptococcal or coccidioidomycosal infections. The 'crescent of air' sign may also be seen in other conditions such as lung abscesses, necrotic tumours, hydatid disease (after cyst rupture) or when blood clots are present in cavities after bleeding. The crescent of air may well be difficult to see on plain X-rays, particularly when there is a significant amount of background pulmonary fibrosis (Fig. 5.2.1).

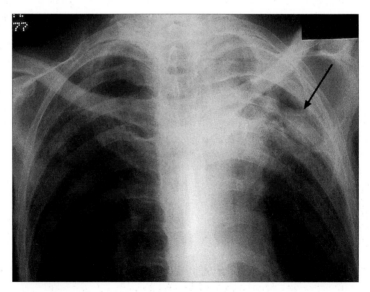

Fig. 5.2.1

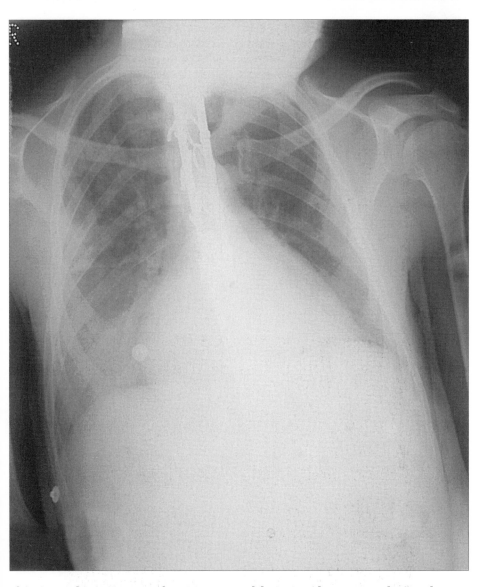

This is a chest X-ray of a 22-year-old man who was admitted to hospital with acute shortness of breath.

A Describe the abnormality and suggest an underlying diagnosis.
B What treatment is indicated?

ANSWER 5.3

A There is marked cardiomegaly and early pulmonary oedema. The patient has had surgical correction of a scoliosis with the insertion of Harrington's rods. The combination of a scoliosis and cardiac failure in a young man suggests Friedreich's ataxia. Patients with this progressive degenerative neurological condition often have a scoliosis and cardiomyopathy as well as pes cavus, ataxia, dysarthria and absent lower limb reflexes.

B Treatment consists of oxygen, diamorphine, diuretics, ACE inhibitors or a nitrate infusion for the pulmonary oedema together with the correction of any dysrhythmia.

A severe thoracic kyphoscoliosis can result in marked deformity of the chest (Fig. 5.3.1) and more significantly can lead to a restrictive lung defect. This may result in right heart failure and polycythaemia secondary to chronic hypoxia. Surgical correction may therefore be indicated in younger individuals with a significant kyphoscoliosis.

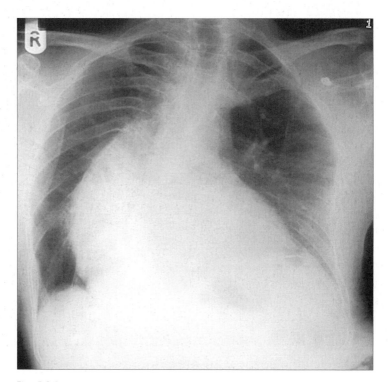

Fig. 5.3.1

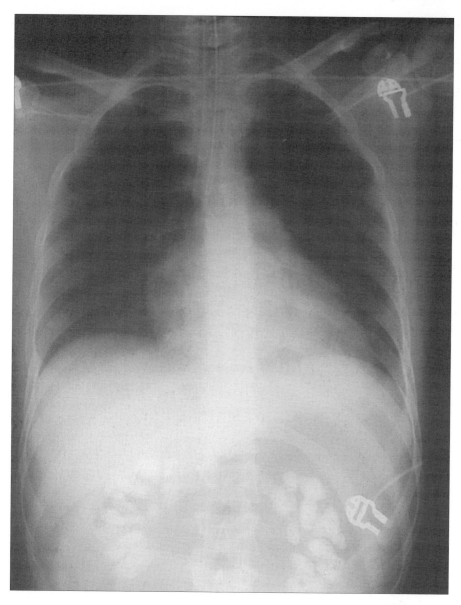

This chest X-ray is of an acidotic 18-year-old man with normal renal function who had a 3-day history of increasing weakness and required ventilation for acute respiratory failure.

A Describe the abnormality and suggest an underlying diagnosis and a cause for his respiratory failure.

B What treatment is required?

ANSWER 5.4

A There are no features to suggest infection, pulmonary oedema or a pneumothorax. However, bilateral nephrocalcinosis is present and in the context of an acidotic patient this suggests an underlying diagnosis of distal renal tubular acidosis. The muscular weakness and respiratory failure is caused by profound hypokalaemia (1.8 mmol/L in this case). It should be noted that a proximal renal tubular acidosis such as occurs in the Fanconi syndrome does not cause nephrocalcinosis. Medullary sponge kidney may also cause nephrocalcinosis but does not cause a disturbance of acid–base balance. Other causes include prolonged hypercalcaemia and primary or secondary hyperoxaluria, but these would only cause an acidosis in the presence of renal failure.

B The acute treatment consists of intravenous potassium and bicarbonate, which must be continued orally in the long term in order to maintain normal potassium and venous bicarbonate levels.

Nephrocalcinosis is secondary to diffuse renal parenchymal calcification and can vary from a few scattered punctate lesions to dense extensive bilateral calcification, which may even be evident on ultrasound (Fig. 5.4.1). Other causes not listed above include hyperparathyroidism, milk alkali syndrome, hypervitaminosis D and sarcoidosis. Renal calcification may also be caused by renal calculi (80% radio-opaque), calcified sloughed renal papillae or tuberculosis, which may give flecks of calcification in multiple granulomata or extensive amorphous calcification in a non-functioning kidney (tuberculous auto-nephrectomy). In addition, 10% of renal tumours and 3% of simple renal cysts exhibit calcification whereas perirenal abscesses or haematomas may eventually calcify.

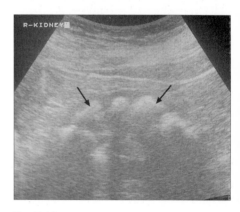

Fig. 5.4.1

QUESTION 5.5

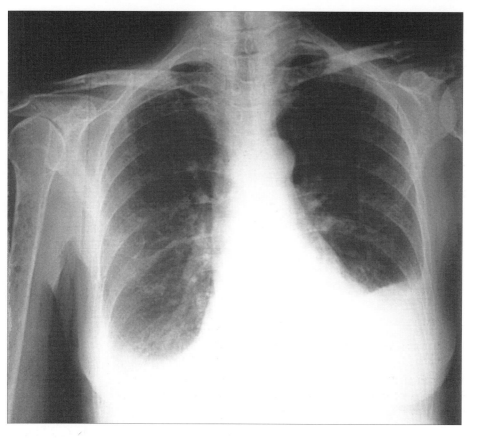

This is the chest X-ray of a 62-year-old woman who was investigated for tiredness, exertional dyspnoea and general 'aches and pains'. She was found to be anaemic, hypercalcaemic and nephrotic.

A Describe the abnormalities.

B Give two possible diagnoses and suggest two causes for the nephrotic syndrome.

C Suggest three useful further investigations.

ANSWER 5.5

[A] There are bilateral pleural effusions but no other evidence of cardiac failure. There are multiple lytic lesions in the skeleton, particularly affecting the right humerus.

[B] Possible diagnoses include multiple myeloma with secondary renal amyloidosis (occurs in 10–20% of patients) or metastatic carcinoma with an associated membranous nephropathy.

[C] Useful further investigations include a bone marrow examination, serum and urine electrophoresis and a renal biopsy.

This case emphasizes the importance of scrutinizing all of the chest X-ray, including a careful assessment of the bones. Hypercalcaemic patients with metastatic carcinoma may be polyuric with a reduced fluid intake and therefore develop prerenal uraemia. Myeloma can affect any part of the skeleton although the classic lytic lesions affect the skull (Fig. 5.5.1), long bones (Fig. 5.5.2) and pelvis (Fig. 5.5.3).

Myeloma may give a similar appearance to osteoporosis when the spine is diffusely affected.

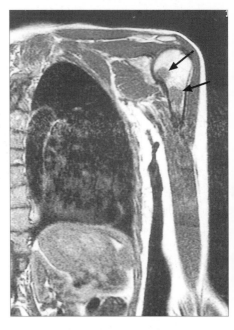

Fig. 5.5.2

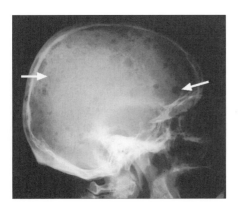

Fig. 5.5.1

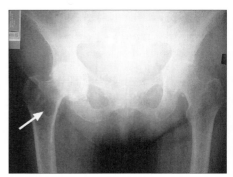

Fig. 5.5.3

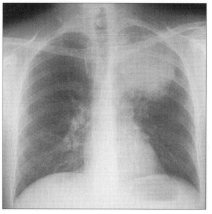

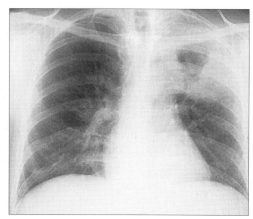

A   **B**

A 36-year-old man was admitted to hospital with a 2-month history of feeling generally unwell with a dry cough and a 1-week history of intermittent fevers. Film A is from the day of admission whereas film B was taken after a 2-week course of intravenous broad spectrum antibiotics. He was still febrile and had developed arthralgias together with a rash over his lower limbs.

A Describe the abnormality in both X-rays and suggest a diagnosis.
B What treatment may be necessary?

A Film A reveals an extensive area of consolidation in the left upper lobe that has undergone cavitation in film B. The lack of a clinical response to a prolonged course of antibiotic therapy coupled with the joint and skin involvement suggests a multisystem disorder which, in the context of a cavitating pulmonary lesion, is most likely to be Wegener's granulomatosis.

B Treatment usually consists of immunosuppression with intravenous methylprednisolone followed by oral prednisolone together with cyclophosphamide, which is usually given orally but may be given as intravenous pulses. Cyclophosphamide is typically changed to azathioprine, which is less myelotoxic, after a few months when the disease is under control. Plasmapheresis may be of some benefit in severe cases such as in patients who are dialysis dependent

at presentation or in those who do not respond well to initial immunosuppression.

Patients with Wegener's granulomatosis may develop pulmonary lesions such as patches of consolidation or nodules that cavitate in about 50% of cases to produce thick-walled lesions. Cavitation is often more evident on a CT scan (Fig. 5.6.1) than on a chest X-ray. Aggressive immunosuppression may, however, lead to impressive radiographic resolution of these lesions (Fig. 5.6.2, same patient post treatment). Pleural effusions are not a prominent feature. Wegener's granulomatosis may occasionally involve the subglottic larynx and proximal trachea, resulting in stridor.

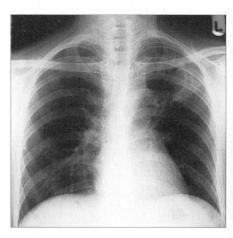

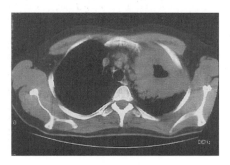

Fig. 5.6.1

Fig. 5.6.2

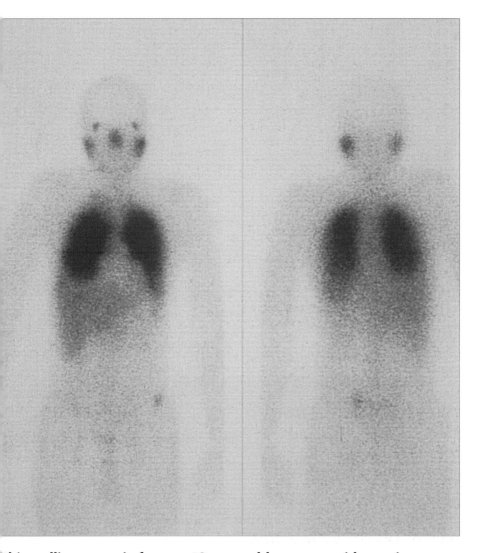

This gallium scan is from a 42-year-old woman with persistent mild hypercalcaemia.

A Describe the abnormality and suggest a diagnosis.
B What clinical features may be present?

ANSWER 5.7

A This gallium scan exhibits a 'snowman' appearance, which is characteristic of sarcoidosis. This appearance is secondary to uptake of gallium by the lacrimal and parotid glands, which are involved in the chronic granulomatous inflammation. Marked uptake in the lungs reflects pulmonary disease and a gallium scan is more sensitive at detecting intrathoracic sarcoidosis than conventional X-rays.

B Possible clinical features include skin involvement (erythema nodosum and lupus pernio), ocular disease (uveitis, lacrimal gland enlargement), uveoparotid fever (Heerfordt's syndrome) and arthralgias. Sarcoidosis may also involve the heart (arrhythmias) and central nervous system (e.g. VII nerve palsy, which may be bilateral).

Sarcoidosis is a multisystem granulomatous disease that may affect almost any tissue or organ. Typically, however, it causes mediastinal lymphadenopathy (Fig. 5.7.1 – effusions are atypical) with or without parenchymal lung involvement. Gallium scans may also be useful in the detection of intra-abdominal abscesses. Although the gallium scan is less sensitive than a labelled white blood cell scan in the detection of acute infective foci it is much more sensitive at detecting chronic inflammation. A gallium scan can also be useful to evaluate the progress of diffuse pulmonary disease during treatment of sarcoidosis. Neurosarcoidosis is best diagnosed by gadolinium-enhanced MRI.

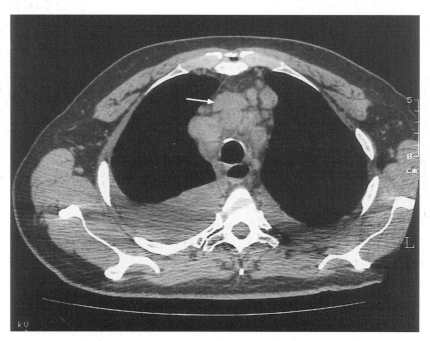

Fig. 5.7.1

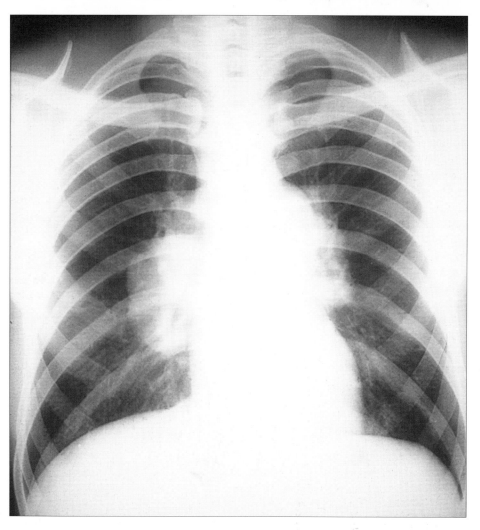

This chest X-ray is of a 29-year-old man and was arranged by his general practitioner in view of the slow resolution of a recent chest infection.

A Describe the abnormality and suggest the two most likely diagnoses.

B What other investigations are indicated and what treatment may be required?

ANSWER 5.8

A There is bilateral hilar lymphadeno-pathy (BHL) with no focal pulmonary pathology. In a young person this is suggestive of either sarcoidosis or lymphoma.

B The patient must be carefully examined for any evidence of lymph-adenopathy or hepatosplenomegaly. A diagnosis of sarcoidosis would be supported by hypercalcaemia, a raised serum angiotensin-converting enzyme (ACE) level, a lymphocytic bronchoalveolar lavage together with noncaseating granulomata evident on a transbronchial biopsy. Pulmonary function tests, renal function and urinalysis are also indicated.

Lymphoma requires a histological diagnosis from a lymph node or bone marrow biopsy and would require chemotherapy and/or radiotherapy depending upon the grade and stage of disease. In the case of sarcoidosis no treatment is required in the absence of lung parenchymal disease but the patient will require regular follow-up and monitoring.

BHL occurs in up to 50% of patients with Hodgkin's lymphoma but the enlargement is usually asymmetrical and often involves all of the hilar and mediastinal lymph nodes (Fig. 5.8.1). BHL may also occur in lymphocytic leukaemias.

Sarcoidosis may be divided into four stages based upon the chest X-ray.

- Stage I is BHL alone.
- Stage II is BHL and diffuse parenchymal involvement.
- Stage III is diffuse parenchymal involvement without BHL (Fig. 5.8.2)
- Stage IV consists of diffuse infiltration, fibrosis and upper lobe cystic and bullous disease.

This staging does provide some indication as to the likelihood of the disease resolving, for example stages I and II resolve in about 55 and 30% of patients,

respectively, without any treatment whereas stage III resolves in less than 5% of patients. Treatment consists essentially of prednisolone although some patients may require additional immunosuppression. Stages II and III are treated if there is evidence of disease progression.

BHL may also be seen in infectious diseases such as tuberculosis, histo-plasmosis, coccidioidomycosis and in viral diseases such as infectious mononucleosis.

Bilateral hilar prominence may also result from enlargement of the pulmonary arteries (e.g. primary arterial hyper-tension, multiple pulmonary emboli and Eisenmenger's syndrome) or veins (e.g. pulmonary venous hypertension secondary to mitral stenosis).

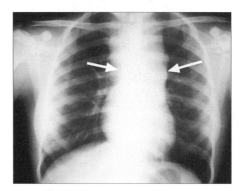

Fig. 5.8.1

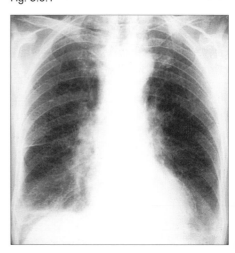

Fig. 5.8.2

QUESTION 5.9

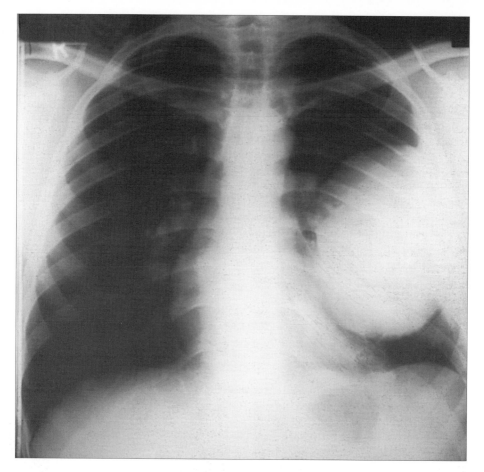

This is a chest X-ray of a 55-year-old dog breeder who complained of a dry cough and some intermittent mild pleuritic discomfort.

A Describe the abnormality and suggest a diagnosis.
B What treatment is available?

A There is a very large well defined opacity in the left mid and lower zone. The remainder of the lung fields are clear. In view of his occupation this lesion may well be a hydatid cyst.

B Treatment consists of surgery to remove discrete lesions and drugs such as praziquantel or mebendazole.

Although hydatid disease has a predilection for the liver it not uncommonly affects the lung where it tends to involve the lower lobes. Cough and pleuritic pain are common symptoms. Serological tests are a useful aid to diagnosis. Hydatid disease may be caused by two different organisms: *Echinococcus granulosus* is contracted from domestic dogs and produces discrete well defined cysts amenable to surgical resection; *Echinococcus multilocularis* is less common and is contracted from wild animals such as foxes. The latter produces more invasive multicystic lesions that are not amenable to surgery.

Other causes of a solitary pulmonary lesion include bronchogenic carcinoma, which may be ill defined and accompanied by lymphadenopathy. This is the most common cause and approximately 30–50% of solitary nodules are malignant. Benign causes include a hamartoma (less than 10% exhibit characteristic popcorn calcification), abscesses, Wegener's granulomatosis (Fig. 5.9.1), infectious diseases such as pneumonia (Fig. 5.9.2 – 'round pneumonia') or tuberculosis (producing the so-called tuberculoma, which often calcifies), histoplasmosis and fungal infections such as coccidioidomycosis. Rarer causes include a solitary metastasis, lymphoma or a rheumatoid nodule.

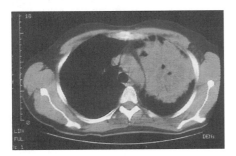

Fig. 5.9.1

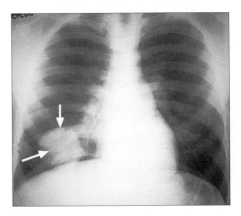

Fig. 5.9.2

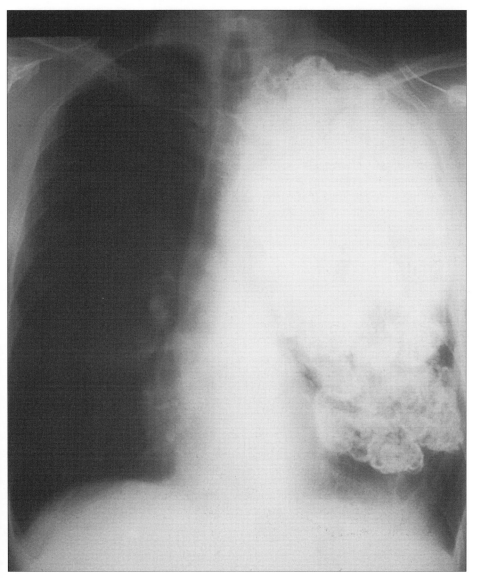

This is a preoperative chest X-ray of a 50-year-old man.

A Describe the abnormality and suggest a diagnosis.
B What treatment is indicated?

A The left hemithorax is almost completely filled with radio-opaque material. This is an example of plombage treatment for previous pulmonary tuberculosis (PTB).

B No treatment is required.

Plombage was a treatment for pulmonary tuberculosis and consisted of filling the space between the chest wall and the infected lung with inert material. This material produced long-lasting collapse of the adjacent tuberculous lung with consequent obliteration of the cavities and would hopefully promote healing.

Plombage treatment avoided the marked chest deformity that accompanied a thoracoplasty (Fig. 5.10.1). Various materials were used, including cellophane (as in this example), plastic packs (Fig. 5.10.2) or plastic lucite spheres. Plombage should not be confused with true upper lobe collapse/consolidation (Fig. 5.10.3). PTB classically produces apical fibrosis and calcification (Fig. 5.10.4).

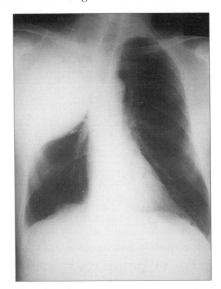

Fig. 5.10.2

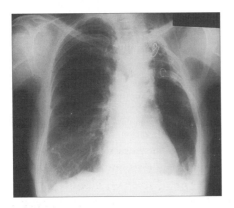

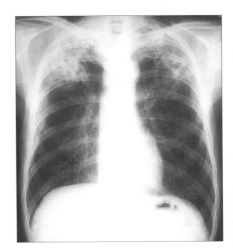

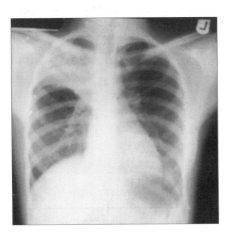

Fig. 5.10.1

Fig. 5.10.3

Fig. 5.10.4

QUESTION 5.11

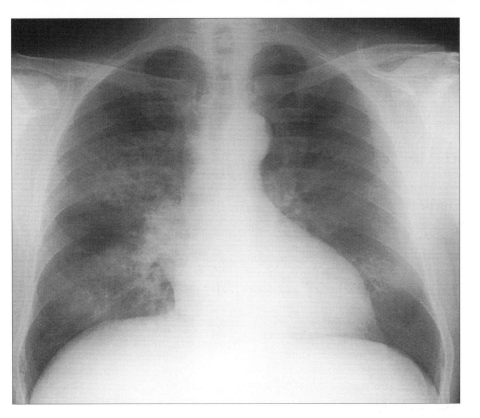

This chest X-ray is of a 54-year-old man who was admitted with a history of increasing shortness of breath. He was hypoxic though afebrile. Jugular venous pressure was not elevated, bilateral basal crackles were audible and mild pedal oedema was present. Investigations revealed the following levels: potassium 7.2 mmol/L, urea 28 mmol/L and creatinine 389 μmol/L; the full blood count and remaining biochemical profile were normal. A Swann–Ganz catheter was inserted and the pulmonary artery capillary wedge pressure (PACWP) was normal and the ECG and cardiac enzymes were unremarkable.

A   Describe the abnormality and give a differential diagnosis.
B   What further investigations are indicated?
C   What treatment is required?

A There is bilateral patchy alveolar shadowing with borderline cardiomegaly. In the context of significant renal failure and a normal PACWP this suggests a diagnosis of pulmonary haemorrhage. Underlying causes might include Goodpasture's syndrome, Wegener's granulomatosis or microscopic polyarteritis. Causes of alveolar haemorrhage such as a bleeding diathesis or idiopathic pulmonary haemosiderosis would not result in renal impairment.

B Further investigations include urine dipstick for haematuria and proteinuria supplemented with urine microscopy for casts, 24-hour urine protein estimation, full immunological screening, including antiglomerular basement membrane antibody levels and antineutrophil cell antibody (ANCA), renal imaging and a renal biopsy. Pulmonary function tests, including a carbon monoxide transfer factor (KCO), are required. The KCO is elevated in alveolar haemorrhage and can be used to monitor the pulmonary status.

C This patient is dangerously hyperkalaemic and requires cardioprotective intravenous calcium together with potassium lowering measures such as intravenous dextrose and insulin and oral or rectal calcium resonium. Intravenous bicarbonate may be cautiously used but not in this patient as it may produce hypervolaemia, which aggravates pulmonary haemorrhage. Dialysis (with minimal heparinization) is indicated if conservative medical measures fail. Treatment for these inflammatory 'pulmonary-renal diseases' consists of immunosuppression with drugs such as cyclophosphamide, azathioprine and steroids. Plasmapheresis is useful in Goodpasture's syndrome unless the patient is anuric, elderly, or has severe crescentic disease.

Pulmonary haemorrhage may occur in the absence of haemoptysis and produces alveolar shadowing that can easily be confused with pulmonary oedema, although radiological signs such as upper lobe blood diversion and Kerley B lines are usually absent. Pulmonary oedema secondary to cardiovascular disease (Fig. 5.11.1) is usually associated with cardiomegaly. It should be noted that pulmonary oedema may be unilateral secondary to postural dependency.

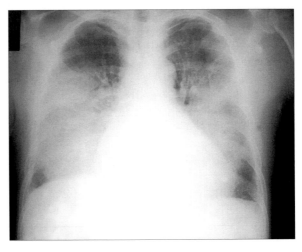

Fig. 5.11.1

QUESTION 5.12

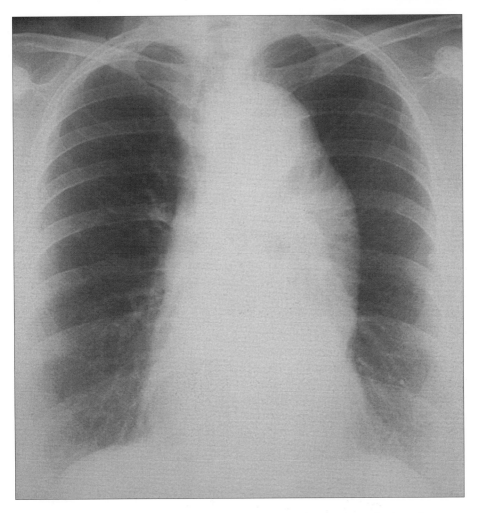

This chest X-ray is of a 64-year-old man who was admitted to hospital with severe acute chest pain.

A Describe the main abnormality and suggest a diagnosis.
B Give two predisposing causes.
C What clinical signs may be present?
D Suggest further investigations and outline treatment.

ANSWER 5.12

A The main abnormality is widening of the superior mediastinum. The history and chest X-ray appearance suggests an acute aortic dissection.

B The most common predisposing causes are hypertension and atherosclerosis. Other causes include connective tissue disorders such as Marfan's syndrome and Ehlers–Danlos syndrome. Syphilitic aortitis is less commonly encountered.

C Clinical signs include asymmetric pulses and blood pressures in the upper limbs together with a pericardial friction rub and the early diastolic murmur of aortic incompetence if the aortic valve is involved. Signs of cerebral or acute mesenteric ischaemia may develop as the dissection progresses.

D Confirmatory investigations include CT or MRI scans together with trans-oesophageal echocardiography; aortography may also be required. Initial treatment consists of analgesia and reduction of blood pressure to normal levels by medical treatment such as intravenous sodium nitroprusside and beta blockers. Acute aortic dissections involving the ascending aorta (type A) require urgent surgery whereas dissections originating beyond the aortic arch (type B) may be treated medically, possibly followed by surgery.

The majority of aortic aneurysms are secondary to atheromatous disease rather than syphilis, although the lattter should be considered. Calcification may be seen in the arterial wall and, if separated from the outer border of the aortic shadow by more than 4 mm, can indicate widening of the aortic wall. Aneurysms may also be secondary to a chronic dissection. A CT scan may exhibit the characteristic 'tennis ball' sign (Fig. 5.12.1) when contrast density differs between the true and false lumens. Causes of a prominent aortic arch include hypertension, atherosclerosis and aortic incompetence as well as the post-stenotic dilatation accompanying aortic stenosis.

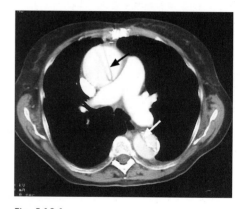

Fig. 5.12.1

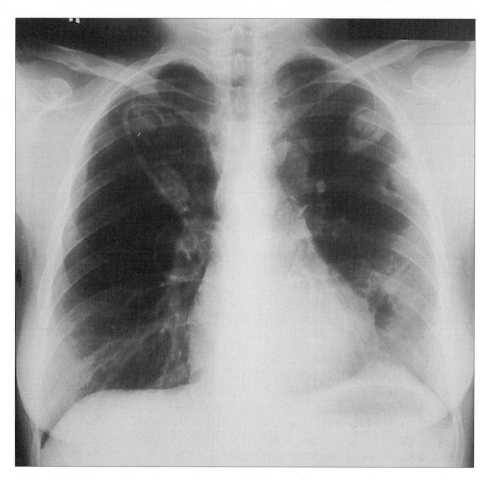

This chest X-ray is of a 32-year-old woman who is receiving chemotherapy for acute myeloid leukaemia and has developed a fever.

A Describe the abnormality and suggest a cause.
B What treatment is required?

ANSWER 5.13

A There is a right Hickman line in situ. There are two peripheral round cavitating lesions in the left upper and mid zones compatible with either pulmonary abscesses or mycetomas. Infection of the Hickman line is a likely source of septic emboli.

B Multiple blood cultures are required to obtain a definitive microbiological diagnosis and treatment instituted with intravenous broad spectrum antibiotics and/or antifungal agents (dependent on the results). The removal of the Hickman line may well be required. The patient must be closely monitored clinically and by echocardiography for the development of endocarditis.

The lesions (Fig. 5.13.1) demonstrate cavitation together with the 'meniscus' or 'air crescent' sign, which may be secondary to inspissated pus or mycetomas. The classic appearance of a pyogenic pulmonary abscess is of a thin-walled cavity with an air-fluid level (Fig. 5.13.2). Abscesses most commonly affect the lower lobes and are often multiple, although they may vary in size. Intravenous indwelling catheters and intravenous drug abuse are predisposing factors.

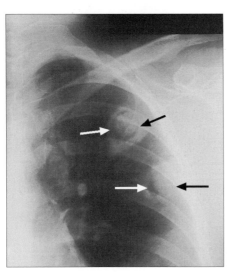

Fig. 5.13.1

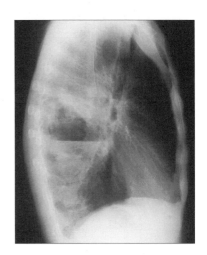

Fig. 5.13.2

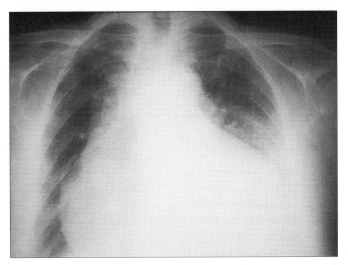

A

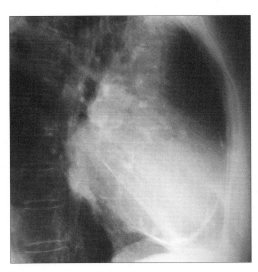

B

Film A is a chest X-ray of a 44-year-old Asian man who was admitted to hospital with a 1-week history of shortness of breath. He also gave a 3-month history of vague ill health with intermittent fevers. Film B is a lateral chest X-ray taken 4 years later when he developed lower limb oedema and abdominal swelling.

A Describe the main abnormality present in both films and suggest a diagnosis.
B What clinical signs may be present and what treatment is available?
C Give three other causes of the radiological appearance seen in film A.

A The main abnormality in film A is gross globular enlargement of the cardiac silhouette whereas in film B there is marked anteroinferior pericardial calcification. The most likely diagnosis in an Asian patient would be a tuberculous pericardial effusion that has subsequently been complicated by pericardial calcification and constrictive pericarditis.

B Symptoms include dyspnoea, weakness and general fatigue. Clinical signs of constrictive pericarditis include chronic oedema, ascites, hepatomegaly (secondary to congestion) with elevation of the jugular venous pressure (JVP). Kussmaul's sign is positive (JVP increases on inspiration). Patients may be treated with diuretics but a surgical pericardiectomy is usually required if the patient is symptomatic.

C See box.

Approximately 50% of patients with chronic constrictive pericarditis have calcified plaques in the thickened pericardium. However, the calcification may not be particularly evident on the posteroanterior chest X-ray (Fig. 5.14.1, same patient and date as 5.14B). Other causes of calcification within the cardiac silhouette include calcification of the coronary arteries (Fig. 5.14.2), valvular calcification or calcification of mural thrombus within an enlarged left atrium or a ventricular aneurysm.

Causes of a pericardial effusion

- Infective pericarditis (usually viral but may be pyogenic)
- Collagen vascular disorders such as SLE
- Pericardial invasion by malignant tumour
- Uraemia
- Myxoedema
- Haemopericardium e.g. after cardiothoracic surgery or secondary to a bleeding diathesis
- Radiation therapy
- Postmyocardial infarction (Dressler's syndrome)

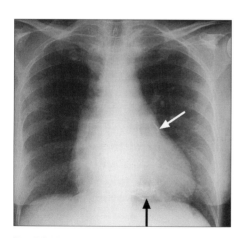

Fig. 5.14.1

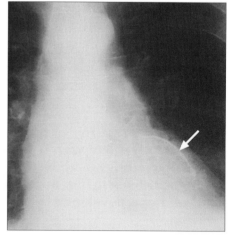

Fig. 5.14.2

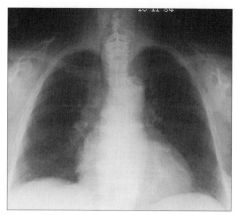

A

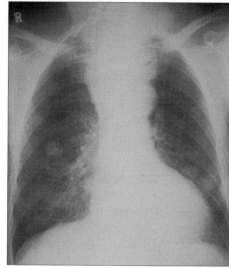

B

Film A is the chest X-ray of a 58-year-old woman who was referred to the medical outpatients department for further investigation of her asthma, which was not responding well to inhaler therapy. Film B is the initial overpenetrated chest X-ray that was taken in the radiology department.

A Describe the abnormality and suggest a diagnosis.
B What treatment is indicated?

A In film A there is marked deviation of the trachea to the right by an upper mediastinal mass. The patient presumably has upper airway obstruction with stridor. Film B demonstrates pulmonary metastases. The most likely diagnosis is carcinoma of the thyroid.

B This patient may have a differentiated, that is papillary or follicular, carcinoma or an undifferentiated anaplastic carcinoma. Initial treatment consists of a surgical total thyroidectomy and thyroxine replacement therapy to maintain a low thyroid-stimulating hormone (TSH) level. Local or distant metastatic disease is present in 4–30% of patients at presentation and may be treated with radioactive iodine if the tumour will concentrate it. Otherwise, external beam radiotherapy is indicated. If histology reveals a medullary carcinoma then the patient should be screened for a multiple endocrine neoplasia type II syndrome. Genetic testing is available and first degree relatives should be screened and offered a prophylactic total thyroidectomy if affected.

There are numerous causes of thyroid gland enlargement such as a simple nontoxic goitre secondary to iodine deficiency, a multinodular toxic goitre or diffuse hyperplasia as well as cancer. A diagnosis can usually be made on the basis of thyroid function tests, and a thyroid ultrasound scan together with a radioisotope scan if indicated. Ultrasound guided fine needle aspiration biopsy (FNABx) or core biopsy can be used to obtain a specific cell type to plan treatment. Aspiration of a large simple cyst may be curative.

Other causes of upper airway obstruction include mediastinal lymphadenopathy secondary to lymphoma or metastatic carcinoma.

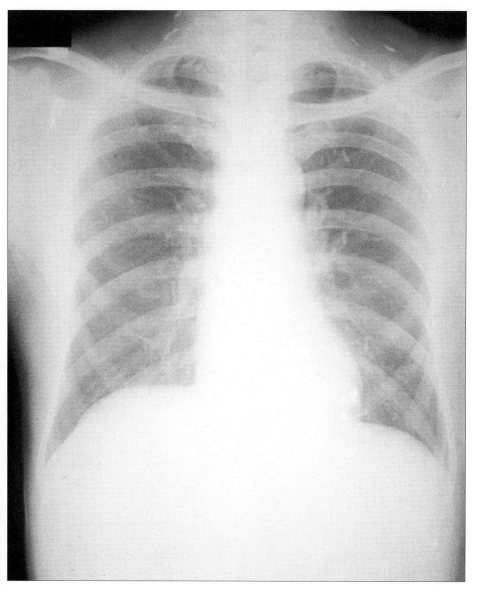

This chest X-ray is from a 21-year-old Nigerian student who was admitted to hospital after an epileptic fit.

A Describe the abnormality and suggest a diagnosis.
B What further investigations are required and what treatment is indicated?

ANSWER 5.16

A There are numerous calcified lesions throughout the soft tissues of the thorax that are aligned in the direction of muscle planes. This patient has cysticercosis. The larvae of the pork tapeworm *Taenia solium* an intestinal infection in humans cause, and poor sanitary habits can lead to, ingestion of the cysticerci, which then results in widespread dissemination throughout the body.

B Serology is useful in confirming the diagnosis. The epilepsy is probably secondary to intracerebral cysts and this patient requires a CT brain scan. Treatment includes anticonvulsants and antihelminthic drugs such as albendazole, praziquantel or mebendazole together with corticosteroids to limit the development of cerebral oedema around the cysts during the treatment period. Cure rate is about 50%. The cysts may be amenable to a surgical excision.

Cysticercosis is an invasive condition and cysts may form in many tissues, including the central nervous system, eyes, striated muscles and subcutaneous tissues. The cysts are most numerous in large striated muscle such as the upper thighs (Fig. 5.16.1). CT scanning is superior for detecting calcified intracranial lesions but MRI scanning is superior for noncalcified cerebral cysts.

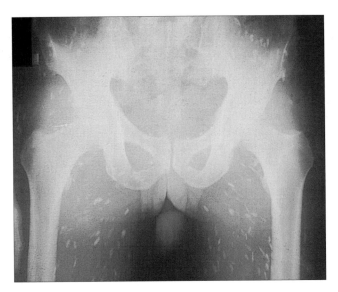

Fig. 5.16.1

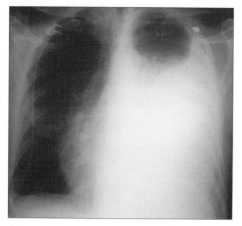

A

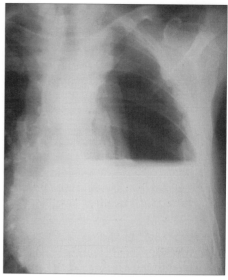

B

Films A and B are of a 57-year-old man and were taken before and after aspiration of pleural fluid. He was admitted to hospital with a short history of increasing shortness of breath.

A Describe the abnormality and suggest a diagnosis.
B Suggest an aetiological factor.

A Film A shows a very large left pleural effusion with mild shift of the mediastinum whereas in film B there is a hydropneumothorax present together with thickening of the parietal pleura (Fig. 5.17.1). This is strongly suggestive of an underlying malignant mesothelioma.

B Asbestos exposure.

A mesothelioma may be benign but the more diffuse malignant lesion associated with exposure to asbestos typically produces a marked pleural effusion that obscures the primary neoplasm. A pleural effusion is rare in the localized benign form. Assessment of the tumour and asso-

ciated malignant invasion of adjacent structures such as bones requires CT scanning (Fig. 5.17.2). Asbestos exposure also causes an increased incidence of bronchial carcinoma and interstitial lung disease. Calcified plaques typically affect the pleura (Fig. 5.17.3).

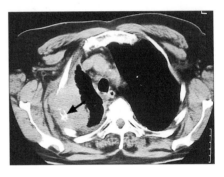

Fig. 5.17.2

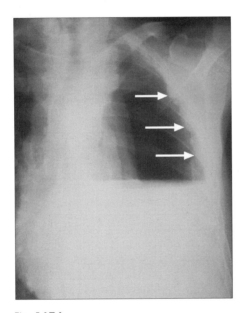

Fig. 5.17.1

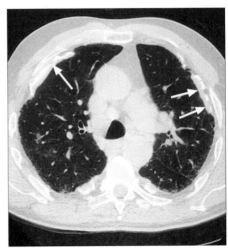

Fig. 5.17.3

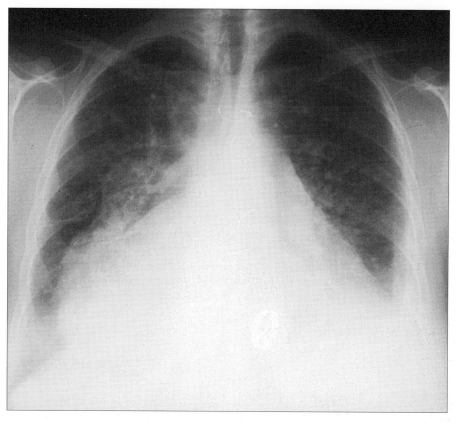

This chest X-ray is of a 67-year-old woman who was admitted to hospital with a short history of increasing shortness of breath associated with episodes of 'shivering'.

A Describe the abnormality and give a differential diagnosis.
B What further investigations are required and what treatment is indicated?

ANSWER 5.18

A There is marked cardiomegaly, upper lobe blood diversion and a left pleural effusion. A mitral valve prosthesis is evident and the splaying of the carina indicates significant left atrial enlargement. This patient is in congestive cardiac failure, which may be the result of numerous causes, including ischaemic heart disease, hypertension and dysfunction of the mitral valve prosthesis.

B Infection must be thoroughly excluded in this patient in view of the history of 'shivering', which is suggestive of a rigor. The patient must be closely examined on a daily basis for any clinical stigmata of infective endocarditis and three sets of blood cultures should be taken immediately and repeated if the patient spikes a fever. Blood tests should include a white blood cell count, C re-active protein, an ESR and serum electrolytes. A transthoracic echocardiogram may be useful but a transoesophageal echocardiogram may be more informative if infective endocarditis is seriously suspected. Treatment for heart failure includes diuretics, ACE inhibitors, vasodilators and possibly digoxin.

There are numerous causes of left atrial enlargement, including mitral regurgitation, mitral stenosis and left to right shunts. Radiological features include elevation of the left main bronchus causing splaying of the carina and a 'double contour' representing the increased density of the enlarged left atrium (Fig. 5.18.1). The left atrium, particularly in mitral regurgitation, may be large enough to cause posterior displacement of the oesophagus and even dysphagia (Fig. 5.18.2).

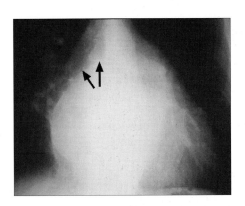

Fig. 5.18.1

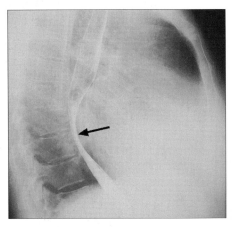

Fig. 5.18.2

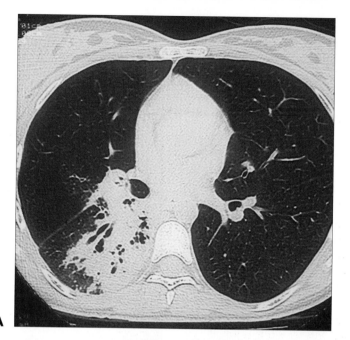

A

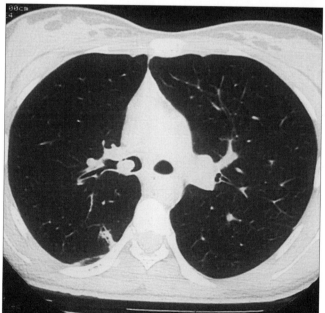

B

Films A and B are CT scans of a 20-year-old woman.

A Describe the abnormality and suggest a diagnosis.
B What further investigations are indicated?

A Film A demonstrates consolidation of the right lower lobe whereas film B reveals the cause – a partially obstructing polyp in the right lower lobe bronchus.

B This patient requires a bronchoscopy and biopsy of the lesion (which proved to be a carcinoid tumour).

Bronchial obstruction may be secondary to benign or malignant tumours as well as inhaled foreign bodies. A flexible or rigid bronchoscopy and biopsy of the lesion is mandatory in these cases. Complete obstruction of the right or left main bronchus results in complete collapse of a lung with a resultant 'white out' and shift of the mediastinum towards the affected side. The main bronchus may come to an abrupt 'cut-off' at the site of the tumour (Fig. 5.19.1). More peripheral lesions can cause segmental collapse or consolidation. Extrinsic compression of a bronchus can also lead to collapse/consolidation as in Fig. 5.19.2 where a large right hilar neoplasm has resulted in right upper lobe collapse/consolidation. Inhaled foreign bodies tend to lodge in the right lower lobe bronchus resulting in right lower lobe collapse (Figure 5.19.3).

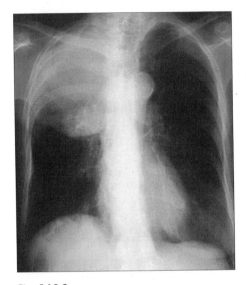

Fig. 5.19.2

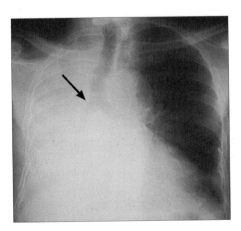

Fig. 5.19.1

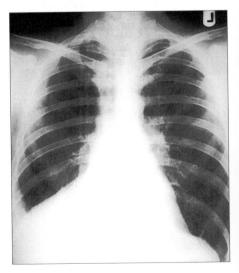

Fig. 5.19.3

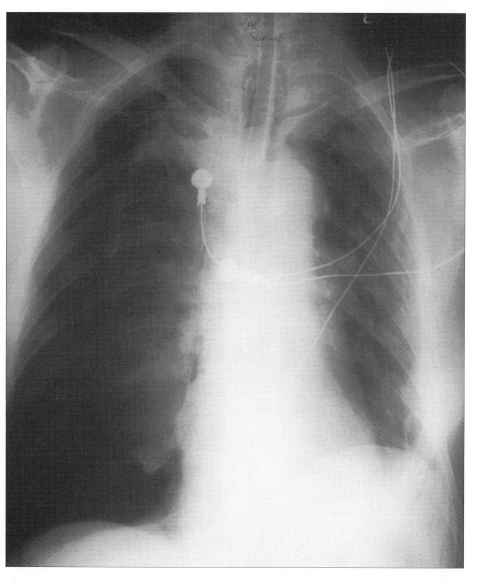

This chest X-ray is of a 39-year-old man in the intensive care department and was taken because of an acute fall in his oxygen saturation.

A Describe the abnormality and indicate what treatment is required.

ANSWER 5.20

A This patient is ventilated. A right pneumothorax is present and is the reason for his deterioration. Insertion of a chest drain is urgently required.

Causes of a pneumothorax include trauma, interstitial lung disease and infections, although the commonest aetiology is spontaneous or iatrogenic. A small pneumothorax may be treated conservatively but a large pneumothorax, particularly when complicating conditions such as chronic obstructive pulmonary disease are present (Fig. 5.20.1), requires drainage. A tension pneumothorax (Fig. 5.20.2) is a medical emergency. A pneumomediastinum (Fig. 5.20.3) may also be spontaneous or iatrogenic but other causes include trauma, asthma, oesophageal rupture and extension of gas from the abdomen.

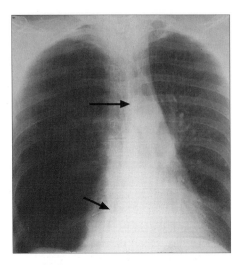

Fig. 5.20.2

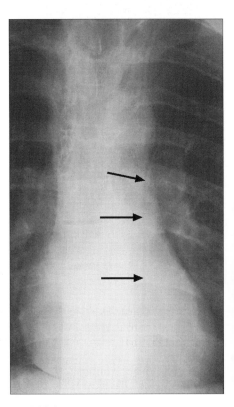

Fig. 5.20.3

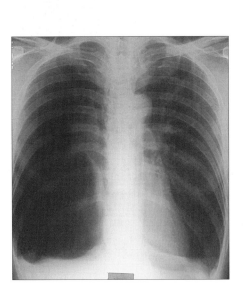

Fig. 5.20.1

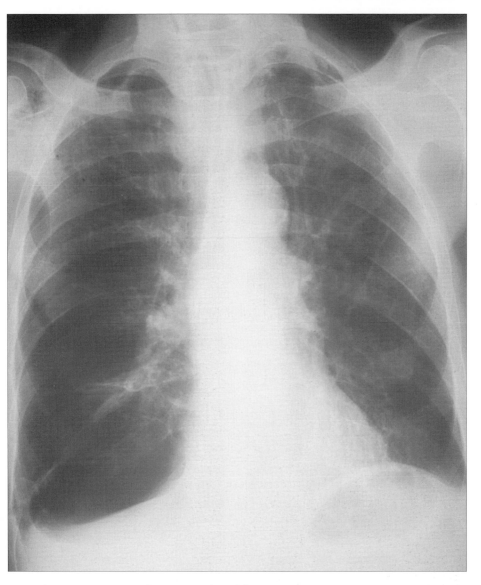

This chest X-ray is of a 59-year-old man.

A Describe the abnormality and suggest a diagnosis.

A There is oligaemia in the right mid and lower zones with associated hyperlucency. This appearance is secondary to the presence of large avascular air spaces or bullae. In view of the diffuse oligaemia in the remaining lung fields this patient has bullous emphysema.

A bulla is defined as an emphysematous air space with a diameter greater than 1 cm. Bullous disease of the lung may occur in the absence of chronic obstructive pulmonary disease or emphysema. Indeed, bullae may be congenital. Bullous disease of the lung usually affects men who only become symptomatic when there is marked compression of the adjacent normal lung parenchyma. It is important to recognize bullae, which may be massive, and not mistake them for a pneumothorax (Figs 5.21.1 – right apical bulla and 5.21.2 – large left bulla). In selected cases a bullectomy may be an option. In bullous disease of the lung the bullae usually occur in the upper lobes whereas in alpha-1-antitrypsin deficiency they predominantly affect the lower lobes. CT scanning usually reveals multiple bullae that are not evident on the chest X-ray. Rupture of a bulla is not an uncommon cause of a pneumothorax or pneumomediastinum in these patients.

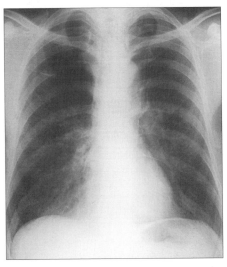

Fig. 5.21.1

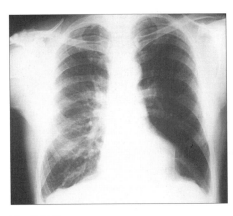

Fig. 5.21.2

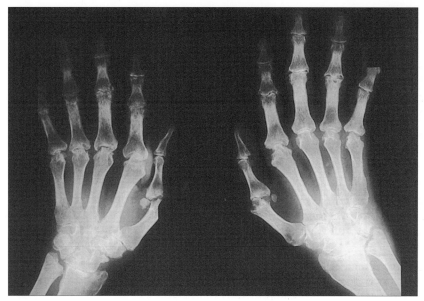

A

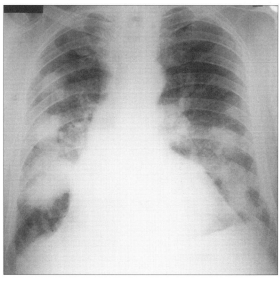

B

Films A and B are of a 59-year-old man who has a longstanding history of arthritis.

A Describe the abnormalities and suggest a unifying diagnosis.
B What physical signs may be present and what treatment is available?

ANSWER 5.22

A Film A demonstrates an inflammatory erosive arthropathy whereas film B demonstrates multiple bilateral opacities of varying size predominantly affecting the mid and lower zones. This patient has rheumatoid arthritis with pulmonary rheumatoid nodules.

B Such patients almost invariably exhibit subcutaneous rheumatoid nodules and may have the typical hand involvement, including ulnar deviation, swan neck and boutonnière deformities. Evidence of skin involvement (ulceration, vasculitis), ocular involvement (scleritis, iritis) or lung involvement (fibrosing alveolitis) may be present. Treatment includes relatively simple measures such as rest, physical therapy and NSAIDs. Ongoing active disease, however, requires treatment with a disease-modifying antirheumatic drug (DMARD) such as hydroxychloroquine (regular fundoscopy), methotrexate (check FBC, LFTs and renal function), sulphasalazine (check FBC and renal function), low-dose prednisolone, gold salts (check FBC and urinalysis) as well as other immunosuppressive agents such as cyclosporin A and azathioprine.

Pulmonary nodules are an uncommon complication of rheumatoid arthritis and they tend to wax and wane according to disease activity. They may undergo cavitation to form thick-walled lesions. Caplan's syndrome is the association of pulmonary rheumatoid nodules with pneumoconiosis. A more serious pulmonary complication is pulmonary fibrosis (Fig. 5.22.1). Hand X-rays may demonstrate bilateral symmetrical involvement of the metacarpophalangeal, proximal interphalangeal and carpal joints with erosive changes, joint space narrowing secondary to destruction of cartilage, periarticular osteoporosis, soft-tissue swelling (joint effusions and hyperplastic synovitis) and joint deformity or subluxation. X-rays of the feet may show similar changes.

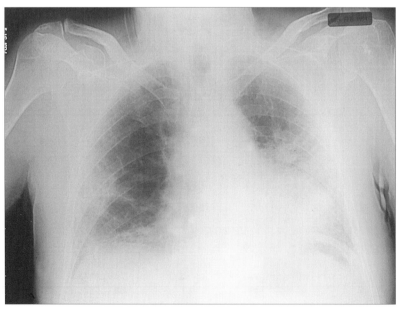

Fig. 5.22.1

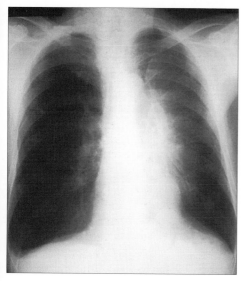 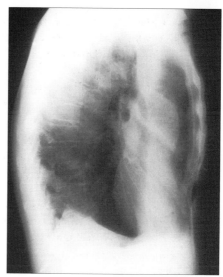

This PA and lateral chest X-ray are of a 50-year-old man who is undergoing investigations for weight loss.

[A] Describe the abnormality.

[B] What further investigations are required?

ANSWER 5.23

A The PA chest X-ray demonstrates mild hyperexpansion of the lung fields. The lateral chest X-ray reveals a wedge-shaped opacity superiorly, which represents a completely collapsed left upper lobe.

B This patient is likely to have a malignant bronchial neoplasm and requires screening blood tests (FBC, calcium, albumin, LFTs etc), sputum cytology and bronchoscopy and biopsy of any intra-bronchial lesion. If a malignant tumour is detected then CT scanning of the chest and imaging of the liver is indicated.

It is important to be able to detect lobar collapse. Left lower lobe collapse classically produces loss of the medial aspect of the left hemidiaphragm with a triangular opacity behind the cardiac silhouette (Fig. 5.23.1). Similarly, right lower lobe collapse produces loss of the medial aspect of the right hemidiaphragm and is not uncommonly seen in patients who have aspirated a foreign body (Fig. 5.23.2). Lobar collapse secondary to mucus plugging (Fig. 5.23.3) or misplacement of an endotracheal tube is an important cause of an acute deterioration in the gas exchange of ventilated patients in the intensive care department. Bronchoscopy and lavage of the affected lobe may be therapeutic in these patients.

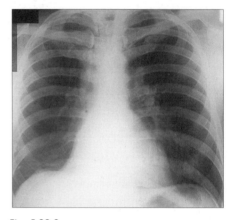

Fig. 5.23.2

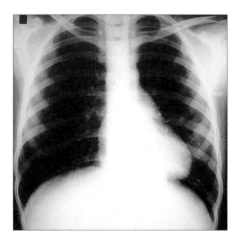

Fig. 5.23.1

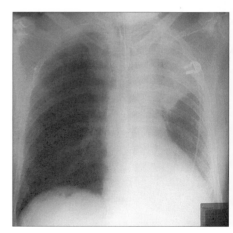

Fig. 5.23.3

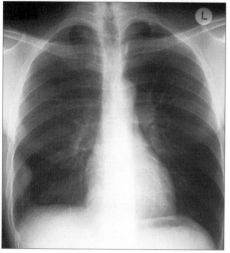

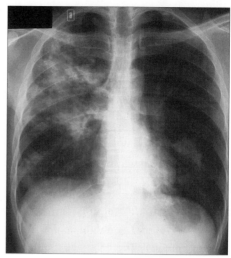

A

B

Film A is a routine chest X-ray of a 35-year-old Chinese man. Film B was taken 4 years later when he was admitted to hospital with a history of fevers, anorexia, weight loss and a dry cough.

A   Describe the abnormalities and suggest a unifying diagnosis.

B   What further investigations and treatment are required?

A Film A is normal apart from an area of pleural thickening in the right lower zone. Film B demonstrates a right upper lobe pneumonia. There is no evidence of cavitation or lymphadenopathy. The most likely diagnosis is tuberculosis. This time delay between primary tuberculosis and the development of overt clinical disease is not unusual.

B This patient requires sputum culture, screening blood tests, skin testing, and possibly bronchoscopy with broncho-alveolar lavage and a transbronchial biopsy in order to obtain a definitive microbiological diagnosis together with drug sensitivities. Combination chemotherapy is usually effective in compliant patients. Contact tracing and assessment is indicated.

Tuberculosis is still prevalent in a number of ethnic groups as well as immuno-suppressed patients and is a cause of significant morbidity. For example, a significant proportion of Asian patients who receive organ transplants develop tuberculosis that may involve a variety of organs (Fig. 5.24.1 – miliary pulmonary tuberculosis) and are often treated with prophylactic isoniazid. Evidence of previous tuberculous infection may be relatively subtle, for example a calcified Ghon focus (Fig. 5.24.2) or gross, such as previous thoracoplasty with extensive pleural calcification (Fig. 5.24.3).

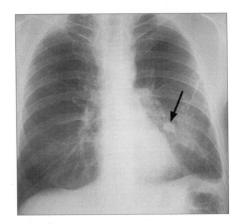

Fig. 5.24.2

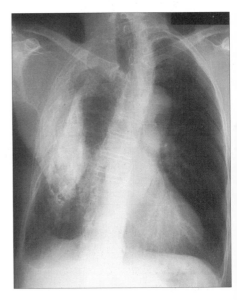

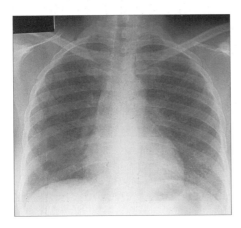

Fig. 5.24.1

Fig. 5.24.3

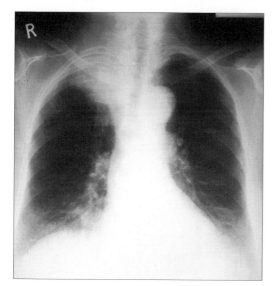

A

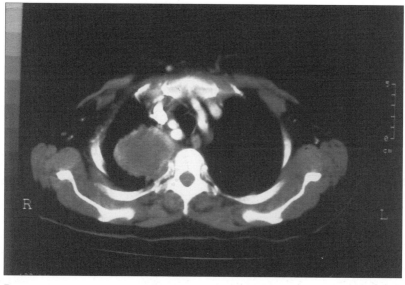

B

Film A is a chest X-ray and film B is a CT scan of a 56-year-old woman who was referred to the medical outpatients department for investigation of paraesthesia and numbness affecting her right forearm.

A Describe the abnormalities and suggest a diagnosis.
B What is the cause of the symptoms?

ANSWER 5.25

A Film A demonstrates an irregular right apical lesion and Film B demonstrates a large solid mass. The diagnosis is a Pancoast tumour.

B The symptoms are secondary to involvement of the lower brachial plexus by the tumour (C8, T1).

CT scanning plays an important role in the management of patients with pulmonary neoplasms and is used to assess lymph node involvement and invasion of adjacent structures such as the mediastinum (Fig. 5.25.1). Although plain chest X-rays are less sensitive they can often detect primary tumours or metastases. The latter may be single (Fig. 5.25.2) or multiple (Fig. 5.25.3), and with or without associated pleural effusions.

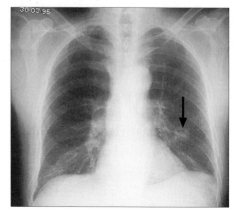

Fig. 5.25.2

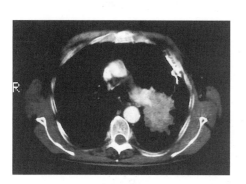

Fig. 5.25.1

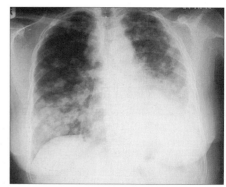

Fig. 5.25.3

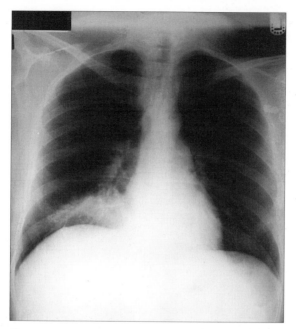

A

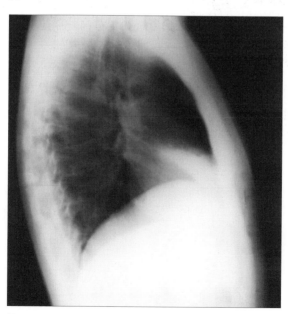

B

Films A and B are PA and lateral chest X-rays, respectively, and are of a 36-year-old man who is a nonsmoker.

A Describe the abnormality and suggest a differential diagnosis.

187

ANSWER 5.26

A These X-rays demonstrate consolidation of the medial segment of the right middle lobe, which is most likely to be secondary to infection. Common organisms that cause a community-acquired pneumonia include *Streptococcus pneumoniae* and *Haemophilus influenzae*; *Mycoplasma pneumoniae*, *Legionella pneumophila*, *Chlamydia pneumoniae* and *Chlamydia psittaci* cause the 'atypical' pneumonias.

The chest X-ray of many patients who present with clinical signs and symptoms of a chest infection simply demonstrate unilateral or bilateral basal shadowing accompanied by loss of the hemidiaphragm (Fig. 5.26.1). In more severe infections, particularly with *S. pneumoniae*, the alveolar shadowing is lobar with an air bronchogram (Fig. 5.26.2). It is important to recognize that the chest X-ray may not reflect the severity of the illness as in Figure 5.26.3, which is normal apart from consolidation of the lingula secondary to psittacosis but the patient was severely hypoxic and nearly required assisted ventilation. Consolidation of the right lower lobe is shown in Figure 5.26.4.

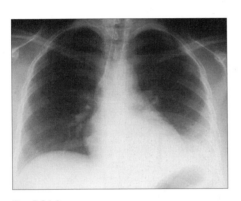

Fig. 5.26.1

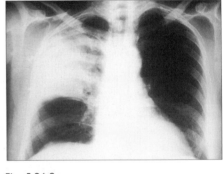

Fig. 5.26.2

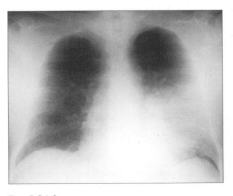

Fig. 5.26.3

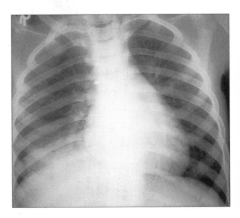

Fig. 5.26.4

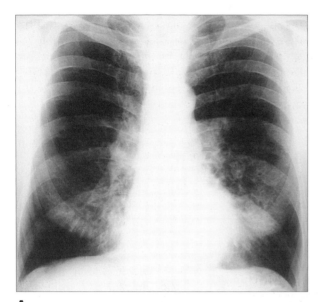

A

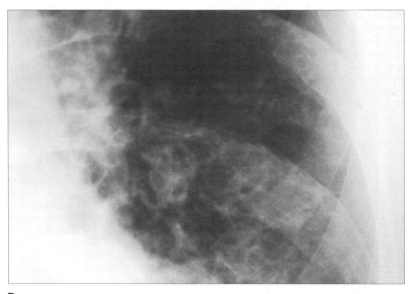

B

Film A is a chest X-ray of a 55-year-old female smoker who was admitted to hospital after an episode of haemoptysis. Film B is a close up of the left mid zone.

A   Describe the abnormality and suggest the most likely diagnosis.
B   What further investigations are indicated?
C   What complications may arise and what treatment is available?

ANSWER 5.27

A The lung fields are mildly hyper-expanded and there is coarse shadowing in the right lower zone and left mid zone. The close up image demonstrates a number of cystic lesions. The most likely underlying diagnosis is bronchiectasis although an occult carcinoma must be excluded.

B A CT scan will determine the extent of disease more accurately and a broncho-scopy is indicated in view of the possi-bility of an incidental bronchial neoplasm.

C Complications of bronchiectasis in-clude systemic amyloidosis, cerebral abscess formation and cor pulmonale. Treatment includes physiotherapy and bronchodilators if indicated together with antibiotics for acute infections. Patients may benefit from alternating courses of oral antibiotics in an attempt to prevent acute exacerbations. Surgery may be indicated for severe recurrent or life-threatening haemoptysis or in patients with localized disease.

Bronchiectasis may be secondary to cystic fibrosis or previous pulmonary infections such as severe pneumonia, tuberculosis or abscesses. In addition bronchiectasis may result from immunodeficiency states such as hypogammaglobulinaemia and com-plicating alpha-1-antitrypsin deficiency. Patients may be clubbed with persistent basal crackles. Chest X-ray findings in-clude crowding of bronchial markings, with the thickened bronchial walls being evident as tramlines. CT scanning demon-strates dilated thick-walled bronchi with cystic spaces that may look like a cluster of grapes (Fig. 5.27.1).

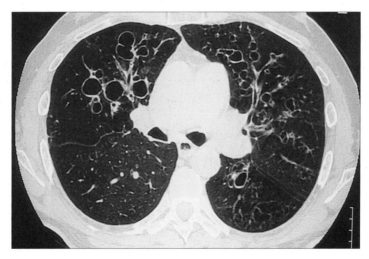

Fig. 5.27.1

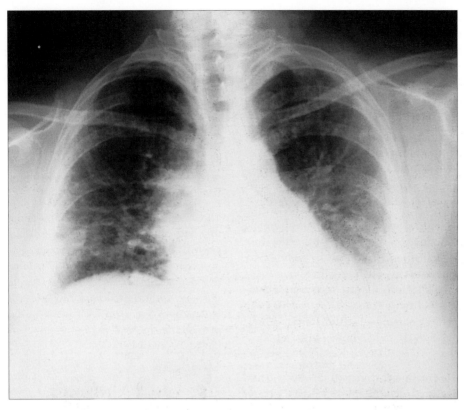

This chest X-ray is from a previously well 52-year-old man who works in an office. He complains of rapidly increasing shortness of breath and cough over several weeks. There is no history of dust exposure or previous lung disease and he is on no medication.

A Describe the abnormality and suggest the most likely diagnosis.
B What are the typical results of pulmonary function tests in this disorder?
C What further investigations are indicated?
D What treatment is available?

A The lung fields are small, with bilateral reticular shadowing more marked on the left. The most likely diagnosis is cryptogenic fibrosing alveolitis (CFA). The rapidity of onset is suggestive of the Hamman–Rich syndrome.

B Pulmonary function testing typically reveals a restrictive ventilatory defect with a significant reduction in the KCO (carbon monoxide transfer factor). Hypoxaemia may be present at rest but is almost invariably present on exercise.

C High resolution CT scanning is indicated together with a bronchoscopy and transbronchial biopsy. It is obviously important to exclude other causes of interstitial lung disease such as bronchiolitis obliterans organizing pneumonia (BOOP), sarcoidosis, bird fancier's lung (Fig. 5.28.1) and lymphangitis carcinomatosis (Fig. 5.28.2).

D Treatment consists of supportive measures, including supplemental oxygen and a trial of corticosteroids, which results in objective improvement in approximately one-quarter of patients. The oxygen saturation on exercise is the most reliable indicator of a response to treatment. Good prognostic features include young age, a short duration of symptoms and a transbronchial or open lung biopsy that exhibits mainly cellular infiltration rather than fibrosis. Cytotoxic drugs such as cyclophosphamide and azathioprine have also been used. In selected patients a heart–lung or single lung transplant may be possible.

The chest X-ray in CFA is usually abnormal and can exhibit a reticular, nodular, reticulonodular or a diffuse ground glass appearance. High resolution CT scanning demonstrates cystic air spaces and reticular infiltrates, which predominantly affect the lower zones (Fig. 5.28.3). CT scanning also provides an accurate guide for open lung biopsy procedures.

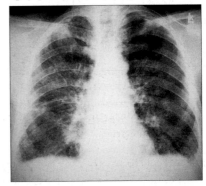

Fig. 5.28.2

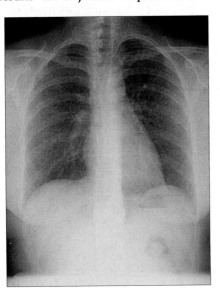

Fig. 5.28.1

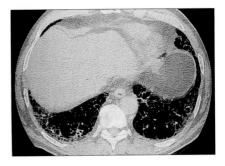

Fig. 5.28.3

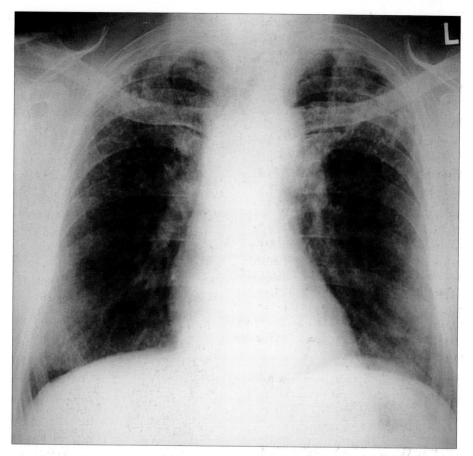

**This is a routine preoperative chest X-ray of a 49-year-old man.
He is a nonsmoker and is asymptomatic.**

A Describe the abnormality and suggest a diagnosis.
B What aspects of the history are important?
C What complications may arise?

A There are small peripheral reticular opacities throughout both lung fields but they are more marked in the upper zones. This suggests silicosis as the most likely diagnosis although coal worker's pneumoconiosis could give a similar appearance.

B The occupational history is important, with particular reference to dust exposure.

C Initially, pulmonary function tests are unaffected but as the disease progresses a mixed obstructive and restrictive picture may develop accompanied by exertional symptoms. It should be noted that there is a higher incidence of tuberculosis in these patients and they should receive a tuberculin skin test.

In silicosis the small silicotic nodules may exhibit punctate calcification whereas the eggshell calcification of hilar lymph nodes is infrequent, although almost pathognomic when present. Other types of stone pneumoconioses may give a similar pattern and the disease may be asymmetrical (Fig. 5.29.1). In complicated silicosis or coal worker's pneumoconiosis cavitation may occur, again affecting the upper lobes more commonly. Progressive massive fibrosis may complicate advanced silicosis or coal worker's pneumoconiosis and is characterized by the presence of large bilateral conglomerate masses that result from the confluence of multiple individual nodules (Fig. 5.29.2).

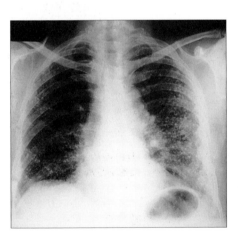

Fig. 5.29.1

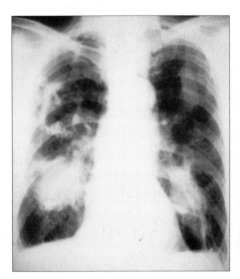

Fig. 5.29.2

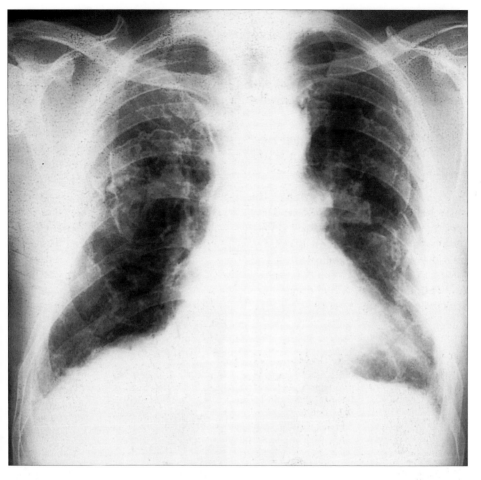

This chest X-ray is of a 60-year-old man who is undergoing investigations for haemoptysis. He has smoked approximately 10 cigarettes per day for 45 years.

A Describe the abnormality and suggest an underlying diagnosis.
B What investigations are indicated?

ANSWER 5.30

A There are fibrotic changes evident throughout both lung fields in association with irregularly shaped pleural plaques in both mid zones. This patient has asbestosis and the haemoptysis and smoking history is strongly suggestive of a bronchial carcinoma.

B This patient requires sputum cytology, a high resolution CT scan of the chest and a fibreoptic bronchoscopy.

Asbestosis affects predominantly the lower lung in contrast to silicosis. X-ray appearances include interstitial fibrosis and pleural thickening and calcification to form the characteristic plaques. Calcified plaques tend to affect the pleura but they may also be evident on structures such as the pericardium (Fig. 5.30.1). Plaques are particularly well demonstrated with high resolution CT scanning, which also demonstrates associated fibrosis (Fig. 5.30.2). Pleural calcification may also arise after the organization of old tuberculous or pyogenic empyemas, haemothoraces and can also be seen in coal worker's pneumoconiosis. Asbestos exposure is associated with a high risk of the later development of mesothelioma and bronchogenic carcinoma; the risk of the latter is dramatically increased by cigarette smoking.

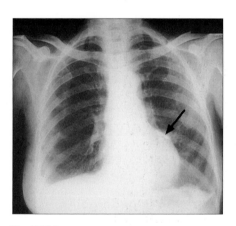

Fig. 5.30.1

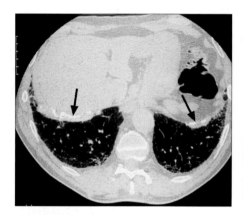

Fig. 5.30.2

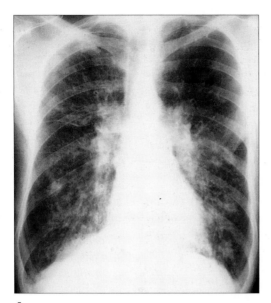

A

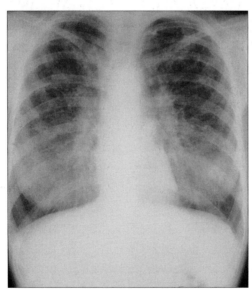

B

Film A is of a 21-year-old man and film B is of his 19-year-old sister.

A   Describe the abnormalities and suggest a disorder that affects both individuals.
B   What is the underlying defect in this disorder?
C   What other clinical manifestations may arise?
D   What treatment is available?

A There is mild hyperinflation of the lung fields in both films with increased interstitial markings, some peripheral rounded opacities and prominent hila secondary to enlarged pulmonary arteries. The family history is strongly suggestive of cystic fibrosis.

B Cystic fibrosis results from a deletion of the CFTR (cystic fibrosis trans-membrane conductance) gene.

C The resultant defective transport of water and chloride across the apical surface of epithelial cells leads to obstruction and damage of exocrine glands by viscid mucus. Apart from chronic lung disease, which may lead to the development of pulmonary hypertension and cor pulmonale, adult patients may also have sinus problems, pancreatic insufficiency, infertility and biliary cirrhosis.

D Respiratory disease may be combatted with chest physiotherapy, inhaled bronchodilators and antibiotics for chest infections according to the results of sputum culture. Recombinant human deoxyribonuclease delivered by aerosol inhalation has been used to cleave the extracellular DNA (derived primarily from neutrophils) that is responsible for much of the increased viscosity of the mucus. In the future, gene therapy may well be effective. Lung or heart–lung transplantation has been used with some success and is the only currently available definitive therapy.

In patients with cystic fibrosis the chest X-ray usually exhibits a coarse interstitial pattern and may well have lobar or segmental collapse superimposed upon it. Thin-walled cysts may develop together with bronchiectasis and bullae. Diffuse peribronchial thickening may appear as a perihilar infiltrate. Pneumothorax is a further complication and is often tolerated poorly.

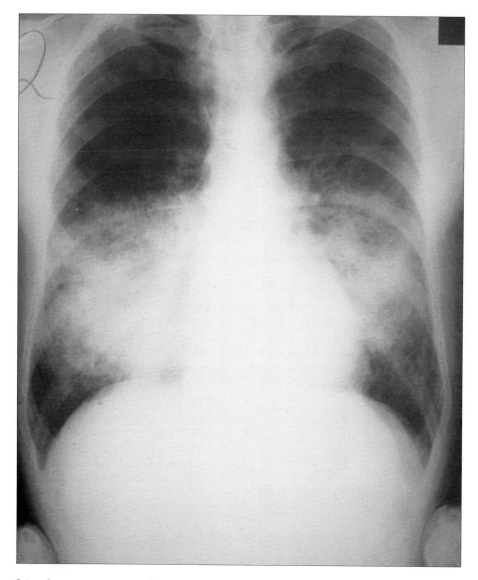

This chest X-ray is of a 33-year-old man who gave a history of mild dyspnoea on exertion for several weeks. There was no history of cough, wheeze, sputum production or haemoptysis. The patient was quite comfortable at rest and examination of the cardiovascular system was unremarkable.

A Describe the abnormalities and give a differential diagnosis. Suggest the most likely diagnosis.

B What is the aetiology of this disorder?

C What treatment is available?

A There is striking bilateral symmetrical alveolar shadowing, which would be consistent with pulmonary oedema or alveolar haemorrhage. However, the absence of evidence of pulmonary hypertension (upper lobe blood diversion or Kerley B lines) and the history makes cardiogenic pulmonary oedema unlikely. Similarly, if this patient had alveolar haemorrhage then he would be unwell. The most likely diagnosis is pulmonary alveolar proteinosis.

B Pulmonary alveolar proteinosis may be a primary disorder or secondary to a variety of conditions, including immunological deficiency states or pulmonary infection with tuberculosis or viruses. There is alveolar deposition of phospholipid material and the diagnosis is based on the appearance of bronchoalveolar lavage fluid, which is milky in appearance and contains PAS-positive lipoproteinaceous material.

C The disease may remit spontaneously or may be progressive. Respiratory symptoms may be ameliorated by bronchial lavage. Patients with pulmonary alveolar proteinosis are susceptible to pulmonary infections with fungi and nocardia.

A symmetrical bilateral pattern of alveolar shadowing may arise in a number of conditions. Cardiogenic pulmonary oedema is the most common and is often associated with cardiomegaly and signs of pulmonary venous hypertension. Note that patients with emphysema and pulmonary oedema may demonstrate a patchy asymmetrical pattern. Noncardiac causes of pulmonary oedema include marked fluid overload secondary to renal failure or possibly over-enthusiastic intravenous fluid replacement, and neurological events such as strokes or inhalation of toxic gases. An almost identical pattern may be seen in widespread pneumonia such as *Pneumocystis carinii* infection, severe aspiration of gastric contents, adult respiratory distress syndrome (Fig. 5.32.1), fat or amniotic fluid embolism, alveolar haemorrhage, increased intracranial pressure, altitude sickness, near-drowning, blunt thoracic trauma or primary pulmonary alveolar proteinosis. Noncardiac causes of pulmonary oedema may well exhibit a normal cardiac size. Bilateral breast implants may occasionally cause confusion (Fig. 5.32.2).

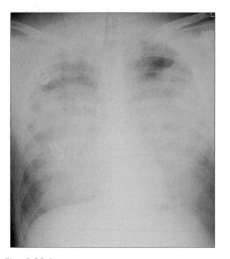

Fig. 5.32.1

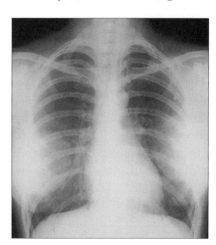

Fig. 5.32.2

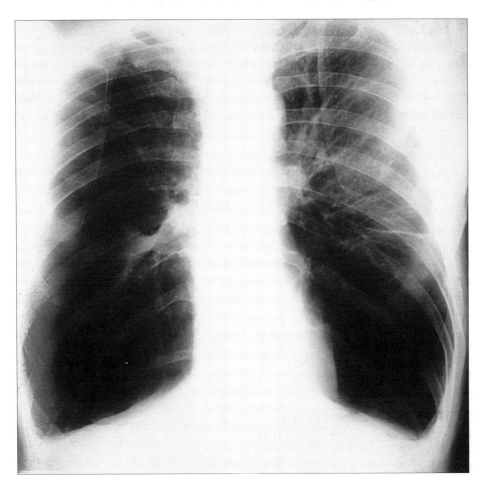

This chest X-ray is of a 29-year-old man who was a mild smoker when a teenager.

A Describe the abnormality and suggest the most likely diagnosis.
B What is the aetiology of this disorder?
C What treatment is available?

A This chest X-ray demonstrates all of the classic features of emphysema with markedly hyperexpanded lung fields, a narrow cardiac silhouette and depressed flattened diaphragms. In addition there is widespread loss of blood vessels in both number and calibre. In a patient of this age the most likely diagnosis is alpha-1-antitrypsin (alpha-1-antiprotease) deficiency.

B Because of the deficiency of alpha-1-antitrypsin the lung is susceptible to protease attack, particularly as a result of smoking. The structural damage to the lung results in parenchymal destruction with the secondary formation of cysts and bullae.

C Patients must not smoke and may benefit from domiciliary oxygen therapy. Intravenously administered recombinant human alpha-1-antitrypsin has been used in selected patients and holds promise for the future but long-term results are not yet available.

Patients with this condition require monitoring of liver function in view of the possible development of cirrhosis. In general, patients with emphysema have less dramatic X-ray appearances (Fig. 5.33.1). It should be noted that respiratory diseases may coexist, as in Figure 5.33.2, which demonstrates the changes of both bullous emphysema and bronchiectasis.

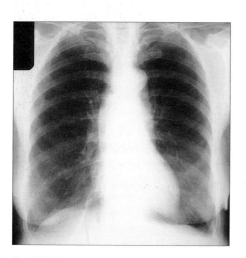

Fig. 5.33.1

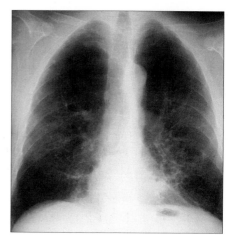

Fig. 5.33.2

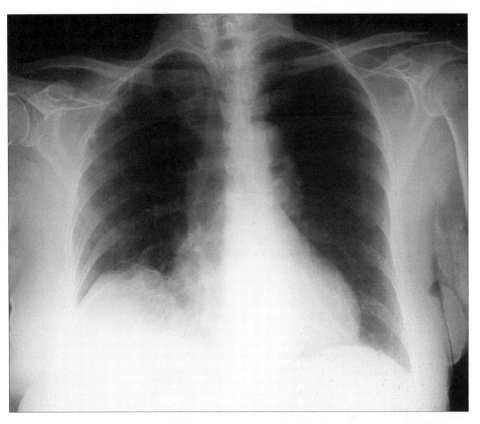

This chest X-ray is of a 46-year-old woman who was admitted to hospital with a history of night sweats and intermittent shivering. On admission she was febrile (39°C) with reduced air entry at the right lung base. There was no stigmata of bacterial endocarditis.

A Describe the abnormality and suggest a diagnosis.
B What further investigations are indicated?

A This chest X-ray does not reveal any obvious thoracic pathology that would account for her symptoms. However, the right hemidiaphragm is markedly elevated (thereby explaining the diminished air entry at the right base) suggesting a subdiaphragmatic diagnosis. The most likely diagnoses are a hepatic or subphrenic abscess.

B An ultrasound is the investigation of choice. It may reveal a hypoechoic hepatic abscess (Fig. 5.34.1) or a collection of fluid in the subphrenic space (Fig. 5.34.2). In both cases aspiration/drainage of the fluid for microbiological culture may be performed under ultrasound control. Multiple blood cultures, liver function tests, full blood count and C reactive protein are indicated.

The subdiaphragmatic regions of a chest X-ray should be scrutinized for abnormal gas patterns, calcification, air-fluid levels

etc. Hepatic abscess may also result in nonspecific right lower zone changes on the chest X-ray (Fig. 5.34.3).

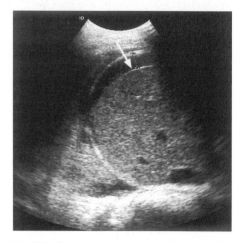

Fig. 5.34.2

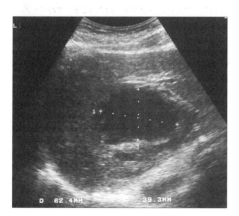

Fig. 5.34.1

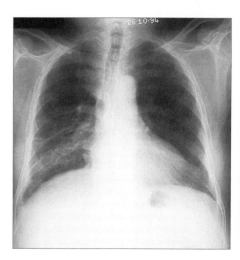

Fig. 5.34.3

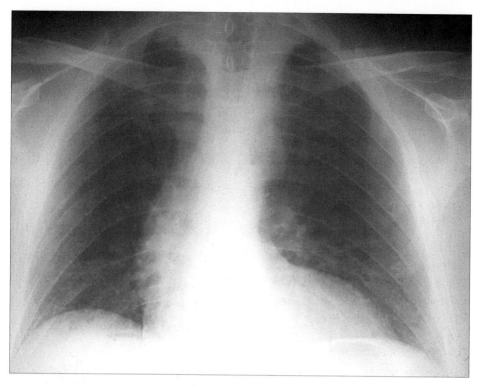

This chest X-ray is of a 31-year-old man who was recently found to be hypertensive.

A Describe the abnormality and suggest a diagnosis.
B What physical signs may be present?
C What treatment is available?

A This chest X-ray exhibits mild cardio-megaly with left ventricular hypertrophy and a small aortic knuckle. In addition, there is notching of the right eighth rib (Dock's sign) (Fig. 5.35.1). This patient has an aortic coarctation.

B Physical signs include weak femoral pulses, radiofemoral delay and a late systolic ejection murmur. There may be prominent arterial pulsations in the neck, and chest wall collateral vessels may be palpable. About one-quarter of patients have a bicuspid aortic valve.

C Surgery is the treatment of choice in young people. Balloon angioplasty may become more prevalent in the future.

Post-stenotic dilatation of the descending aorta may be evident in such patients. The aortic knuckle may be enlarged in hypertensive patients and may become aneurysmal (Fig. 5.35.2). Calcification of the aortic knuckle is common in the elderly. Calcification may be more promi-nent in aortic aneurysms (Fig. 5.35.3 – post-thoracic trauma).

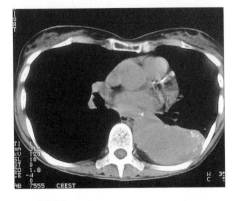

Fig. 5.35.2

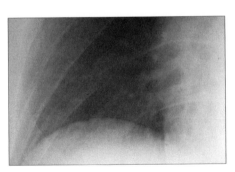

Fig. 5.35.1

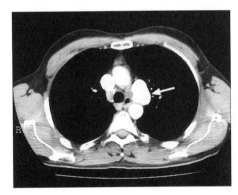

Fig. 5.35.3

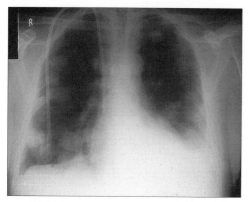

A

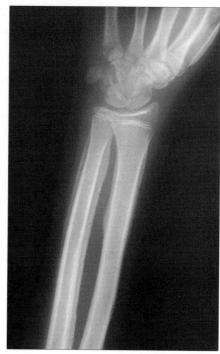

B

Films A and B are of a 46-year-old man who is on haemodialysis.

A Describe the abnormalities and suggest a diagnosis.
B What physical sign may be present?

ANSWER 5.36

A There is a right Francis catheter in situ (vascular access for haemodialysis) together with multiple metastases and a left pleural effusion. Film B demonstrates an exuberant periosteal reaction that affects the radius and ulna. This patient has hypertrophic pulmonary osteoarthropathy, which is most likely secondary to disseminated bronchogenic carcinoma.

B Clubbing is almost invariably present in these patients.

The periosteal reaction may be florid and if markedly irregular may resemble 'candle wax', although in early disease the appearance may be more subtle (Fig. 5.36.1). Hypertrophic pulmonary osteoarthropathy is most commonly found in patients with bronchogenic carcinoma but other causes include pulmonary metastases from extrathoracic primary tumours or mesothelioma. Non-neoplastic causes include chronic suppurative lung diseases (pulmonary abscesses, bronchiectasis or empyema), cystic fibrosis, cyanotic cardiac disease and gastrointestinal diseases such as cirrhosis or inflammatory bowel disease.

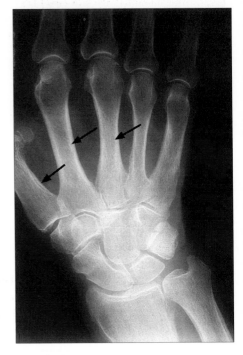

Fig. 5.36.1

QUESTION 5.37

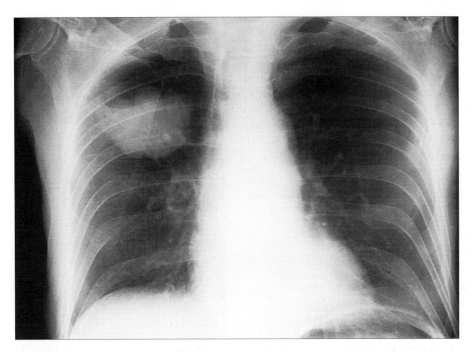

This chest X-ray is of a 57-year-old man who presented to his general practitioner with polyuria, polydipsia and increasing headaches. A preoperative chest X-ray performed 6 months earlier was normal.

A Describe the abnormality and suggest a diagnosis and two causes for his polyuria.

B What further investigations are indicated?

A There is a large solitary rounded lesion in the right upper lobe. The most likely diagnosis is a bronchogenic carcinoma. The polyuria may be secondary to hypercalcaemia or diabetes insipidus. The history of headaches suggests secondary infiltration of the pituitary gland, leading to antidiuretic hormone (ADH) insufficiency.

B The specific gravity of the urine should be checked (usually < 1.006) and routine haematological and biochemical tests performed, particularly calcium. Diabetes mellitus must be excluded. An MRI of the pituitary and hypothalamus is required to exclude a mass lesion. Cranial and nephrogenic diabetes insipidus may be differentiated by a supervised water deprivation test (modest fluid restriction only if nephrogenic disease is strongly suspected). Administration of desmo-

pressin reduces the thirst and polyuria in cranial diabetes insipidus.

This patient had a carcinoma of the lung (Fig. 5.37.1) with metastatic disease involving the pituitary gland (Fig. 5.37.2, arrow) where a further deposit is seen in the left Sylvian fissure (Fig. 5.37.2, arrowhead). Approximately one-third of metastases to the pituitary gland cause diabetes insipidus whereas it is relatively uncommon in pituitary adenomas, occurring in about 1% of patients.

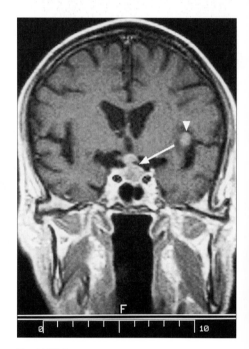

Fig. 5.37.2

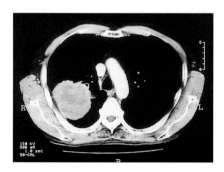

Fig. 5.37.1

QUESTION 5.38

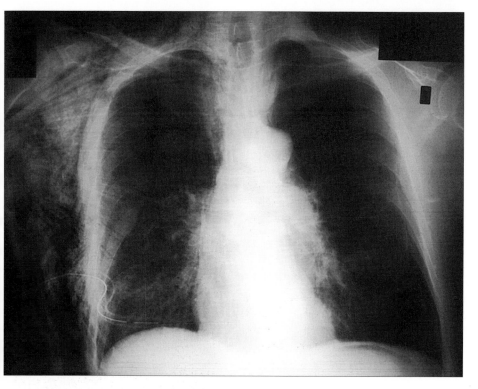

This chest X-ray is of a 29-year-old man.

A   Describe the abnormalities and suggest a diagnosis.

A There are bilateral pneumothoraces with gross, mainly right-sided surgical emphysema. A right basal chest drain has been inserted.

The surgical emphysema (Fig. 5.38.1) in this patient may be secondary to trauma or a misplaced chest drain. Air within the soft tissues may be readily identifiable on plain X-rays in conditions such as gangrene (Fig. 5.38.2). Other sites where the presence of air is abnormal includes the pericardium (Fig. 5.38.3) or the pleural space (Fig. 5.38.4).

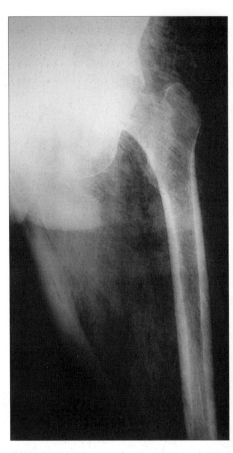

Fig. 5.38.2

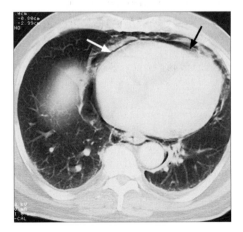

Fig. 5.38.1

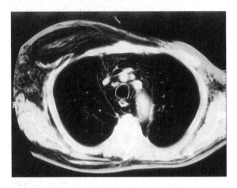

Fig. 5.38.3

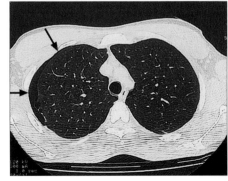

Fig. 5.38.4

QUESTION 5.39

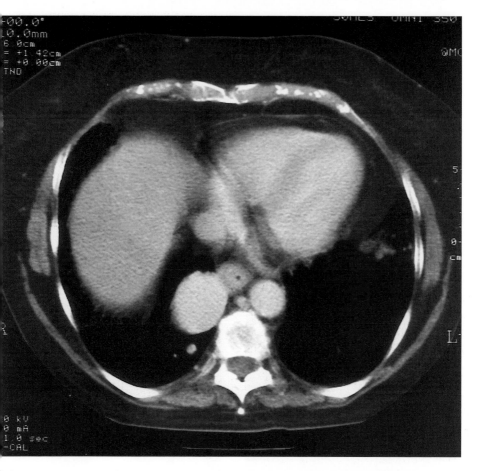

This CT scan (with contrast) is of a 32-year-old nonsmoking woman who is hypoxic at rest and has secondary polycythaemia.

A Describe the abnormalities and suggest a diagnosis.
B What treatment is available and what are the potential complications of treatment?

A There are multiple rounded uniformly enhancing lesions in the lung fields. In the context of the history this suggests multiple pulmonary arteriovenous malformations as a cause for her symptoms.

B Right-to-left shunting in the lungs may occur through small (microvascular) or large pulmonary arteriovenous malformations. The microvascular lesions are not amenable to treatment but the larger lesions may be treated by selective embolization. The main risk of the procedure is if the embolic material were to pass through the arteriovenous malformation into the systemic arterial circulation and block an end artery, resulting in, for example, a cerebral infarction.

Pulmonary angiography is required in these patients to determine the number, location and size of the shunts. Because of the potential risks embolization is usually restricted to the largest shunts. Polycythaemia may also be secondary to neoplasia, particularly renal cell carcinoma (Fig. 5.39.1, left renal mass), but may also occur in small cell carcinoma of the lung (Fig. 5.39.2).

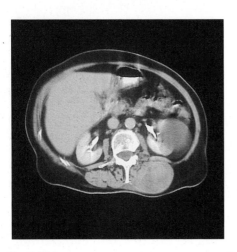

Fig. 5.39.1

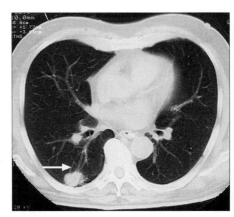

Fig. 5.39.2

INDEX